LIFETIME WEIGHT CONTROL PATIENT COUNSELING

Third Edition

By
Nancy Gustafson, MS, LRD

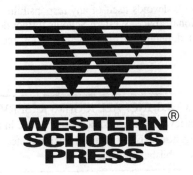

WESTERN SCHOOLS® PRESS

21 Bristol Drive

South Easton, MA 02375

1-800-618-1670

ABOUT THE AUTHOR

Nancy Gustafson, MS, LRD, is a registered dietitian and freelance medical writer. She has authored or co-authored numerous articles and three books on diet and health for both lay and professional audiences. She earned a BS in nutrition from the University of Minnesota and an MS in nutrition with a minor in journalism from the University of Maryland. She has served as a nutritionist with the US Department of Agriculture, as a clinical dietitian with the University of Maryland Hospital in Baltimore, and as publications coordinator for the Metabolic Research Group at the University of Kentucky in Lexington. As an outpatient dietitian at Carle Clinic in Urbana, IL, she specialized in weight control and developed behavior modification, very low-calorie diet, and individualized weight management programs.

Based on the book *Lifetime Weight Control: Patient Counseling, Second Edition,* by Jean Holliday, RN, and Mary Stein.

Managing Editor: Aimee Squires, RN, MA

Graphic Artist: Kathy Johnson

Typesetter: Gwen Nichols

ISBN: 1-878025-45-7

IMPORTANT: Read these instructions *BEFORE* proceeding!

Enclosed with your course book you will find the FasTrax answer sheet. Use this form to answer all the final exam questions that appear in this course book. If you are completing more than one course, be sure to write your answers on the appropriate answer sheet. Full instructions and complete grading details are printed on the FasTrax instruction sheet, also enclosed with your order. Please review them before starting. *If you are mailing your answer sheet(s) to Western Schools, we recommend you make a copy as a backup.*

ABOUT THIS COURSE

A "Pretest" is provided with each course to test your current knowledge base regarding the subject matter contained within this course. Your "Final Exam" is a multiple choice examination. **You will find the exam questions at the end of each chapter.** Some smaller hour courses include the exam at the end of the book.

In the event the course has less than 100 questions, mark your answers to the questions in the course book and leave the remaining answer boxes on the FasTrax answer sheet blank. Use a black pen to fill in your answer sheet.

A PASSING SCORE

You must score 70% or better in order to pass this course and receive your Certificate of Completion. Should you fail to achieve the required score, we will send you an additional FasTrax answer sheet so that you may make a second attempt to pass the course. Western Schools will allow you three chances to pass the same course…*at no extra charge!* After three failed attempts to pass the same course, your file will be closed.

RECORDING YOUR HOURS

Please monitor the time it takes to complete this course using the handy log sheet on the other side of this page. See below for transferring study hours to the course evaluation.

COURSE EVALUATIONS

In this course book you will find a short evaluation about the course you are soon to complete. This information is vital to providing the school with feedback on this course. The course evaluation answer section is in the lower right hand corner of the FasTrax answer sheet marked "Evaluation" with answers marked 1–25. Your answers are important to us, please take five minutes to complete the evaluation.

On the back of the FasTrax instruction sheet there is additional space to make any comments about the course, the school, and suggested new curriculum. Please mail the FasTrax instruction sheet, with your comments, back to Western Schools in the envelope provided with your course order.

TRANSFERRING STUDY TIME

Upon completion of the course, transfer the total study time from your log sheet to question #25 in the Course Evaluation. The answers will be in ranges, please choose the proper hour range that best represents your study time. You MUST log your study time under question #25 on the course evaluation.

EXTENSIONS

You have 2 years from the date of enrollment to complete this course. A six (6) month extension may be purchased. If after 30 months from the original enrollment date you do not complete the course, *your file will be closed and no certificate can be issued.*

CHANGE OF ADDRESS?

In the event you have moved during the completion of this course please call our student services department at 1-800-618-1670 and we will update your file.

GUARANTEE

If any continuing education course fails to meet your expectations or if you are not satisfied in any manner, for any reason, you may return it for an exchange or a refund (less shipping and handling) within 30 days. Software, video and audio courses must be returned unopened.

Thank you for enrolling at Western Schools!

WESTERN SCHOOLS
P.O. Box 1930
Brockton, MA 02303
(800) 618-1670

LIFETIME WEIGHT CONTROL
PATIENT COUNSELING

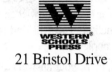

WESTERN®
SCHOOLS
PRESS

21 Bristol Drive
South Easton, MA 02375

Please use this log to total the number of hours you spend reading the text and taking the final examination (use 50-min hours).

Date	Hours Spent
9 - 3	3 hrs

TOTAL

Please log your study hours with submission of your final exam. To log your study time, fill in the appropriate circle under question 25 of the FasTrax® answer sheet under the "Evaluation" section.

Please choose the answer that represents the total study hours it took you to complete this 30 hour course.

A. less than 25 hours   C. 29–32 hours

B. 25–28 hours   D. greater than 32 hours

LIFETIME WEIGHT CONTROL PATIENT COUNSELING

WESTERN SCHOOLS' NURSING
CONTINUING EDUCATION EVALUATION

Instructions: Mark your answers to the following questions with a black pen on the "Evaluation" section of your FasTrax® answer sheet provided with this course. You should not return this sheet. Please use the scale below to rate the following statements:

A	**Agree Strongly**	**C**	**Disagree Somewhat**
B	**Agree Somewhat**	**D**	**Disagree Strongly**

The course content met the following education objectives:

1. Identified some key issues in weight management.

2. Explained some of the genetic, physiological, environmental, and psychological reasons why obesity is so prevalent in our society.

3. Identified the many ways that obesity and marked overweight contribute to serious medical problems and recognized how obesity can affect societal attitudes and body image.

4. Described the key elements of a comprehensive assessment of the obese patient.

5. Indicated appropriate weight management choices for patients with different degrees of obesity and medical risk.

6. Recognized the nutritional components of a balanced diet and described how macronutrients and micronutrients help maintain overall good health.

7. Identified characteristics of a balanced, low-calorie diet and indicated how to select an appropriate calorie level and nutrient composition.

8. Described food-related behaviors and activities that can improve adherence to diet plans.

9. Identified dietary considerations for special groups of patients.

10. Described the benefits of regular exercise and specified guidelines for exercising safely.

11. Identified factors that help patients achieve life-long dietary and exercise changes.

12. The content of this course was relevant to the objectives.

13. This offering met my professional education needs.

14. The information in this offering is relevant to my professional work setting.

15. The content of this course was appropriate for home study.

16. The course was generally well written and the subject matter explained thoroughly? (If no please explain on the back of the FasTrax instruction sheet.)

17. The final examination was well written and at an appropriate level for the content of the course.

Please complete the following research questions in order to help us better meet your educational needs. Pick the ONE answer which is most appropriate. Proceed directly to question #25 to log in your course study time if you do not want to answer the following questions.

18. For your LAST renewal did you take more Continuing Education contact hours than required by your state, if so, how many?

    A. 1–15 hours   C. 31 or more hours

    B. 16–30 hours   D. No, I only take the state required minimum

19. Do you usually exceed the contact hours required for your state license renewal, if so, why?

    A. Yes, I have more than one state license   C. Yes, for professional self-interest/cross-training

    B. Yes, to meet additional special association Continuing Education requirements   D. No, I only take the state required minimum

20. What nursing shift do you most commonly work?

    A. Morning Shift (Any shift starting after 3:00am or before 11:00am)   C. Night Shift (Any shift starting after 7:00pm or before 3:00am)

    B. Day/Afternoon Shift (Any shift starting after 11:00am or before 7:00pm)   D. I work rotating shifts

21. What was the SINGLE most important reason you chose this course?

    A. Low Price   C. High interest/Required course topic

    B. New or Newly revised course   D. Number of Contact Hours Needed

22. Where do you work? (If your place of employment is not listed below, please leave this question blank.)

    A. Hospital   C. Long Term Care/Rehabilitation Facility/Nursing Home

    B. Medical Clinic/Group Practice/ HMO/Office setting   D. Home Health Care Agency

23. Which field do you specialize in?

    A. Medical/Surgical   C. Pediatrics/Neonatal

    B. Geriatrics   D. Other

24. For your last renewal, how many months BEFORE your license expiration date did your order your course materials?

    A. 1–3 months   C. 7–12 months

    B. 4–6 months   D. Greater than 12 months

25. **PLEASE LOG YOUR STUDY HOURS WITH SUBMISSION OF YOUR FINAL EXAM.** Please choose which best represents the total study hours it took to complete this 30 hour course.

    A. less than 25 hours   C. 29–32 hours

    B. 25–28 hours   D. greater than 32 hours

CONTENTS

PRETEST

Begin by taking the pretest. Compare your answers on the pretest to the answer key (located in the back of the book). Circle those test items that you missed. The pretest answer key indicates the course chapters where the content of that question is discussed.

Next, read each chapter. Focus special attention on the chapters where you made incorrect answer choices. Study questions are provided at the end of each chapter so you can assess your progress and understanding of the material.

1. Compared with the adult average, which of the following groups of Americans has a lower prevalence of obesity?

    a. while males
    b. black females
    c. minority populations
    d. older individuals

2. With increasing body mass index, death rate:

    a. remains unchanged
    b. increases in a J-shaped curve
    c. increases linearly
    d. decreases linearly

3. About what percentage or all Americans are overweight?

    a. less than 15%
    b. 15 to 20%
    c. 25 to 30%
    d. over 40%

4. The change from a nation of hunters to an agriculture society led to:

    a. no noticeable change in average weights
    b. depletion of food stores
    c. opportunity for obesity to develop
    d. greater protein intake

5. Compared with normal-weight individual, most obese persons eat:

    a. about 1,000 more calories daily
    b. about 500 more calories daily
    c. slightly more calories daily
    d. about the same or fewer calories daily

6. Obesity increases the risk of what type or cancer?

    a. skin cancer
    b. colon cancer
    c. thyroid cancer
    d. liver cancer

7. How early in life does atherosclerosis begin?

    a. after age 40
    b. after age 35
    c. in the 20s and 30s
    d. in adolescence

8. Which of the following is least relevant in obtaining a health history from an obese individual?

    a. the patient's weight at birth
    b. age of onset of the patient's obesity
    c. experience with previous weight loss attempts
    d. incidence or obesity in mother or father

9. Which of the following can be a physical sign of poor nutrition?

    a. smooth, slightly moist skin
    b. psychological stability
    c. reddish pink mucous membranes in oral cavity
    d. dry, thin hair

10. Weight loss is achieved when:

    a. The balance of calories taken in and calorie expended does not affect weight loss
    b. Calories taken in are greater than calories expended
    c. Calories taken in are balanced with calories expended
    d. Calories taken in are fewer than calories expended

11. Which of the following is not an important element of behavior modification?

    a. stimulus control
    b. self-monitoring
    c. cognitive restructuring
    d. psychotherapy

12. For which of the following groups is weight loss contraindicated?

    a. children
    b. young adults
    c. older adults
    d. weight loss is not contraindicated for any group

13. Protein should provide what percentage of total calorie intake in a balanced diet?

    a. 12–20%
    b. 25–28%
    c. 30–38%
    d. 50% or more

14. Protein, carbohydrate, and fat are referred to as:

    a. micronutrients
    b. macronutrients
    c. meganutrients
    d. complex nutrients

15. Most women will lose about one pound weekly on how many calories daily?

    a. 800
    b. 1,200
    c. 1,500
    d. 1,800

16. Which food exchange list do potatoes belong in:

    a. starch/bread list
    b. vegetable list
    c. fat list
    d. combination list

17. How many cents out of every food dollar does the average American spend away from home?

    a. 20
    b. 30
    c. 40
    d. 50

18. Under the new labeling regulations, food manufacturers can use terms like "low" and "reduced":

    a. in an unrestricted manner
    b. only if they apply for permission first
    c. food manufacturers can no longer use such terms
    d. only if their products meet the strict definitions for these terms

19. For an individual trying to lose weight, which of the following would probably be the best choice at a fast food restaurant?

   a. a plain burger
   b. a salad with dressing
   c. a baked potato with cheese
   d. a fish sandwich

20. A desirable blood cholesterol level for adults is:

   a. less than 180mg/dl
   b. less than 200mg/dl
   c. 200–239mg/dl
   d. less than 240mg/dl

21. Which type of cholesterol increases risk of coronary heart disease the most?

   a. very low-density lipoprotein cholesterol
   b. low-density lipoprotein cholesterol
   c. intermediate-density lipoprotein cholesterol
   d. high-density lipoprotein cholesterol

22. For a person weighing 160 pounds, adding a 45-minute walk three days weekly would produce a yearly weight loss of about:

   a. 2 pounds
   b. 9 pounds
   c. 18 pounds
   d. 26 pounds

23. Regular physical activity:

   a. raises levels of high-density lipoprotein cholesterol
   b. raises blood glucose levels
   c. increases appetite
   d. depresses endorphins

24. which of the following best describes effective obesity treatment?

   a. Obesity is a disease that can only be cured with caloric restriction and exercise.
   b. Obesity is a chronic disease that requires long-term treatment.
   c. Obesity results from faulty food behaviors which must be addressed during treatment.
   d. Tthe primary treatment for obesity is increased physical activity.

25. All of the following are elements of a successful weight maintenance program except:

   a. setting realistic weight loss goals
   b. not expecting perfect adherence to diet
   c. exercising regularly
   d. adhering to a rigid diet

PREFACE

Many experts believe that obesity is the number one health problem in America today, affecting one-quarter to one-third of our population. Unfortunately, the social and psychological implications of obesity are all too obvious, but obesity isn't just a matter of cosmetic concern—it's a matter of life and death.

Obesity is an independent risk factor for coronary heart disease, the number one cause of death in America. Being overweight also increases risk for high blood pressure, high blood cholesterol, diabetes, gallbladder disease, gout, and some types of cancer. To put it more directly, the death rate increases proportionately to degree of obesity.

Because of those risks, the National Heart, Lung, and Blood Institute recently launched the "Obesity Education Initiative" to educate health professionals and the public on the causes, consequences, and treatments of obesity.

Dieting has become a national habit. Today we can't pass a bookstore, turn on a television set, or pick up a newspaper without seeing or hearing about a new diet. Over 50 percent of all adults and an alarmingly high percentage of school-aged children report having dieted at some point.

Americans spend billions of dollars on weight reduction aids, clinics, spas, organized weight reduction programs, diet books, diet pills, special foods, and health clubs.

Why are Americans spending so much of their time, energy, and money dieting? Because Americans are more overweight than ever before and because of the sad truth that most diets don't work. Some researchers estimate that 90 percent of all patients who lose more than 25 pounds in a diet program regain these pounds within three years.

Does this mean we should give up dieting and be content to remain obese? No, but perhaps we should re-examine our goals. Studies show that even modest weight losses of 10 to 20 pounds can significantly improve health and reduce high blood pressure, diabetes, high blood cholesterol levels, and risk for coronary heart disease.

Dr. George Blackburn, a well-known obesity expert with Deaconess Hospital in Boston, states that "just a 10-pound loss per overweight person in the United States would reduce the national health bill by $100 billion (Blackburn & Kanders, 1987)." Further, the health and psychological effects of repeatedly losing and regaining large amounts of weight are unclear.

Today the emphasis for weight control has shifted from quick-fix diets to long-term weight control and obesity prevention. Obesity is a chronic disease that requires life-long management.

This book will help nurses assist patients in their pursuit of lifetime weight control by emphasizing permanent healthy eating and lifestyle changes. Nurses, along with physicians, registered dietitians, and other health care professionals, can offer effective intervention strategies to help patients lose weight and keep it off.

The first three chapters explore the prevalence, causes, and consequences of obesity. The chapters that follow outline weight management strategies from a nursing process perspective.

Chapter 4 describes assessment of the obese patient, and Chapter 5 gives an overview of alternative weight management options. Chapters 7 through 9 focus on intervention plans that foster healthy low-fat eating for life—not temporary, crash diets.

Chapter 10 describes the critical role of exercise intervention in weight management. Finally, Chapter 11 discusses the goal of intervention efforts—permanent, weight loss maintenance.

CHAPTER 1

THE CHALLENGE OF LIFETIME WEIGHT CONTROL

CHAPTER OBJECTIVE

After reading this chapter, you will be able to identify some of the key issues in weight management.

LEARNING OBJECTIVES

After studying this chapter, you will be able to:

1. Specify trends in the prevalence of obesity in men, women, and minorities.
2. Recognize the health risks of obesity as well as the benefits and risks of weight loss.
3. Discuss important elements of effective intervention strategies.

INTRODUCTION

At any given time, over 20 million Americans are dieting—that's about one in every three people. Dieting has become a national practice and way of life for many people in recent years. Consider these facts:

- About 25 to 30 percent of all Americans are overweight
- About 50 percent of all women have gone on a diet
- About 25 percent of all men have gone on a diet
- Crash diets have a 2 to 5 percent success rate

Although adults 35 to 49 years of age make up the largest group of dieters, even young children are aware of our society's diet mentality. In a recent survey of children in rural Iowa, 40 percent of fourth-graders reported having gone on a diet, 60 percent wished they were thinner, and 80 percent knew of a family member who had dieted (Gustafson-Larson & Terry, 1992).

With this great preoccupation with thinness, the diet industry is big business in America. According to a congressional house subcommittee report on "Deception and Fraud in the Diet Industry" (1990), Americans spend over $33 billion each year trying to lose weight; by 1995 they are projected to spend more than $50 billion trying to lose weight.

This chapter examines some of the reasons why Americans are spending so much time, money, and energy dieting. Chapter 1 will discuss the prevalence of obesity in America and give a perspective on its historical development. It will provide a brief overview of the types of obesity and associated health risks. Finally, Chapter 1 will summarize the complexity of obesity treatment.

PREVALENCE OF OBESITY IN AMERICA

Obesity is the most common nutrition-related problem in America, affecting nearly 44 million people. Based on data from the National Center for Health Statistics (1989), 27 percent of adult women and 24 percent of adult men are overweight. Gortmaker et al. (1987) reports that one in four children in America are overweight.

The prevalence of obesity in the United States has doubled since the early 1900s (Brownell, 1983). Between 1974 and 1980, the number of obese Americans has increased 20 percent (Skelton & Skelton, 1992). Even more alarming is the 54 percent increase of obese children 6 to 11 years of age and the 39 percent increase of obese children 12 to 17 years of age over approximately this same time period (Gortmaker et al., 1987).

As illustrated in Figures 1.1 and 1.2, obesity is more common among older age groups, women, and minority populations. Thirty-nine percent of women and 25 percent of men between the ages of 65 and 74 years are overweight. The prevalence of obesity increases steadily up to age 55 in men and up to age 65 in women.

Several minority groups are particularly at risk for obesity (McGinnis & Ballard-Barbash, 1991). Obesity is more common among black and Mexican-American men and women than among white men and women. Black women have the highest incidence of overweight, affecting nearly 50 percent of the population (Kumanyika, 1987). Between 45 to 55 years of age, obesity is twice as prevalent in black women as in white women. Socioeconomic status also affects obesity prevalence. Men with incomes above the poverty line are more likely to be obese, whereas the opposite is true for women (Skelton & Skelton, 1992).

HISTORICAL PERSPECTIVE

For 95 to 99 percent of our history, humans lived exclusively as hunters and food gatherers (Stuart & Davis, 1972). The change from hunting and gathering to an agricultural society has had important implications for obesity.

The genetic tendency to store excess calories as fat may once have been advantageous. Ironically, as Brown and Konner (1987) have noted, what is now a metabolic problem may once have been a superior survival trait among certain peoples. That is, some persons use less of their food energy stores to produce heat (thermogenesis) and thus have a more efficient energy system. Unfortunately, with easy access to foods, what was originally a boon to the survival of our species may now be a hazard to our health.

Because food shortages were the norm for all humans under natural conditions, natural selection favored persons who could effectively store calories when food was plentiful, to carry them through times when food was scarce. Brown and Konner (1987) have reported that food scarcities would occur at least every two to three years and that fat stores would be depleted in about 75 percent of people. Women with greater energy reserves have a selective advantage over their leaner counterparts, and are better able to withstand the stress of food shortages not only for themselves but for their fetuses or nursing infants as well. Women also characteristically have a slower release of peripheral fat than men, which once was a necessity for reproductive fitness and survival. Thus, many individuals may have had the ability to become obese, but never the opportunity to do so, at least until recent times.

Isolated cases of obesity have been recognized for thousands of years. An early Stone Age statuette

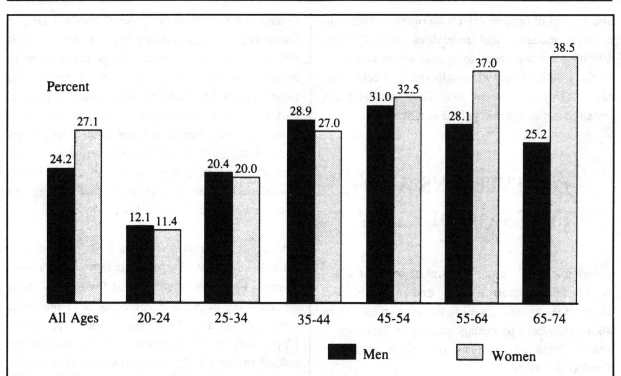

Figure 1.1 Prevalence of overweight according to sex and age.

Source: National Center for Health Statistics. Najjar, MR, Rowland, M. (1987). Anthropometric reference data and prevalence of overweight, United States, 1976–80. *Vital Health Statistics* (11) 238:1–73.

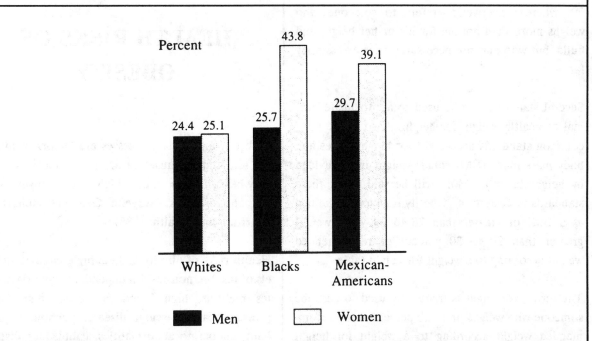

Figure 1.2 Prevalence of overweight among blacks, whites, and Mexican-Americans by sex.

Source: National Center for Health Statistics. Najjar, MR, Rowland, M. (1987). Anthropometric reference data and prevalence of overweight, United States, 1976–80. *Vital Health Statistics* (11) 238:1–73; and National Center for Health Statistics. Najjar, MR, Kuczmarski, RJ. (1989) Anthropometric reference data and prevalence of overweight for Hispanics: 1982–84. *Vital Health Statistics* (11) 239: 1–106.

and symbol of fertility depicts an obese woman with a large abdomen and pendulous breasts (Bray, 1992b). Obesity began to appear more commonly in the English upper classes in the eighteenth and nineteenth centuries, but only since the 1940s has obesity been widely recognized as a health hazard.

DEFINITIONS AND TYPES OF OBESITY

Everyone has a certain amount of body fat which is necessary for storing energy and supporting and cushioning organs. Obesity, however, refers to an abnormally large percentage of body fat that impairs health (National Institutes of Health Consensus Conference, 1985).

Strictly speaking, the terms *overweight* and *obese* are not the same. Obesity refers to an excess of body fat, whereas overweight refers to someone who weighs more than normal for his or her height and build, but who may not necessarily have excess body fat.

Several standards can be used to approximate normal or healthy weight for height. Two of the most common standards are weight for height tables and body mass index (BMI equals weight in kg divided by height in m^2). More will be said about these standards in Chapter 4. Obesity is generally defined as a BMI of greater than 28 to 30, or a weight greater than 20 to 30 percent of recommended weight according to a weight for height table.

The term overweight is frequently used to describe someone who weighs up to 20 percent above recommended weight according to a weight for height table. Someone weighing up to 20 percent more than the standard may not be overfat, just well muscled.

Consider, for example, a National Football League linebacker. A well-muscled football player who is 6'4" tall could easily weight 240 pounds and be in excellent health. Yet according to height and weight charts he would be 40 pounds overweight. Although he is overweight, he is not overfat or obese, just well muscled. Since most of us are not professional football players, however, most Americans who are classified as overweight are also obese. Therefore the terms overweight and obesity are used interchangeably in this book.

Another consideration is where fat deposits are located in the body. Fat deposits in the upper body (around the waist, flank and abdomen) are more metabolically active than fat deposits in the lower body (thigh and buttocks) (Bjorntorp, 1991). Upper body obesity is associated with greater health risks than lower body obesity (Despres et al., 1990). Women tend to have more lower body obesity, whereas men tend to have more upper body obesity.

HEALTH RISKS OF OBESITY

Obesity and dietary excesses are factors in five of the ten leading causes of death in America—coronary heart disease, stroke, high blood pressure, cancer, and diabetes (Surgeon General's Report on Nutrition and Health, 1988).

Health risks of obesity include high, circulating levels of insulin, non-insulin dependent (type II) diabetes mellitus, high blood fat levels, high blood pressure, cardiovascular disease, pulmonary problems, endocrine abnormalities, gallbladder disease, cancer, musculoskeletal disorders, obstetric complications, and increased surgical risk (Van Itallie, 1979; National Research Council, 1989).

Dr. George Blackburn, head of a center for the study of nutrition and medicine at Deaconess Hospital in Boston, states that people endanger their health when they weigh as little as 15 percent more than they should. Bray (1992) recently proposed a classification system for determining medical risks from obesity based on body mass index (BMI). A BMI of:

- 20 to 25 indicates very low medical risks,
- 25 to 30 indicates low risk,
- 30 to 35 indicates moderate risk,
- 35 to 40 indicates high risk, and
- greater than 40 indicates very high risk.

In a recent review, Sjostrom (1992) notes that people with a BMI of 35 or more (corresponding to a weight of 230 pounds or more for a person 5'8" tall) have at least twice the mortality rate compared with people in the normal weight range.

Age of onset of obesity may also affect health risks later in life. Dr. Aviva Must (1992) interviewed individuals who were originally studied between 1922 and 1935. The average age of participants at follow-up was 73 years. Men who were overweight as adolescents had about twice the death rate, especially from coronary heat disease, as men who were lean as adolescents. Women who were overweight as adolescents did not appear to have a higher death rate than women who were lean as adolescents; they had a higher incidence of arthritic problems.

Overall death rate increases with increasing body weight (National Research Council, 1989). The statistical relationship between overall mortality and body mass index is usually *J-shaped*, meaning a higher death rate at slightly under mean body weight and steadily increasing rates as body weight increases (Van Italiie, 1992). This J-shaped curve also applies to mortality from cardiovascular diseases, cancer, diabetes, hypertension, gallbladder disease, and osteoporosis (Bray, 1985).

HEALTH BENEFITS OF WEIGHT LOSS

Even modest weight loss of about 10 percent of body weight (20 pounds for someone weighing 200 pounds, for example) improves health and decreases medical problems in 90 percent of obese patients (Blackburn, 1987). Modest weight loss improves heart function, blood pressure, blood sugar control, sleep disorders, and blood lipid profiles. Such weight losses also decrease the need for medication, hospitalizations, and postoperative complications (Robison, 1993).

In a review of the effects of weight loss in obese patients, Goldstein (1992) noted significant health improvements in patients with type II diabetes, high blood pressure, high blood cholesterol levels, and cardiovascular disease when they lost about 10 percent of body weight. Such modest losses also appeared to increase longevity in obese individuals.

Weight loss decreases the incidence and severity of both hypertension and type II diabetes. Recent studies have even suggested weight loss may prevent the onset of these diseases for some people (National Institutes of Health, 1992). Weight loss also reduces or eliminates the need for medication in some people with diabetes or high blood pressure.

Cardiovascular risk directly decreases with weight loss. Data from the Framingham study suggest that a 10 percent decrease in body weight corresponds to a 20 percent decrease in risk of developing coronary artery disease (Ashley, 1974). Modest weight losses also decrease cardiovascular risk in women, even when they still remain obese (Tremblay, 1992).

Besides physical benefits, weight loss in very obese persons has been associated with improved functional status, reduced work absenteeism, less pain, and greater social interaction.

HEALTH RISKS OF WEIGHT LOSS

Although the health benefits of weight loss are well documented, weight loss can also have some negative effects (National Institutes of Health, 1992). Persons on very strict weight loss diets often report fatigue, hair loss, and dizziness. Weight loss in persons who are only slightly overweight leads to greater loss of lean body mass (muscle tissue) than in severely overweight individuals. Dieting may also increase the risk of binge eating.

The health effects of repeated weight loss and regain, called *weight cycling*, are unclear (Robison, 1993). Some studies suggest that weight cycling may change the way the body handles energy.

A study by Steen and colleagues (1988) showed that wrestlers who repeatedly lost and regained weight had slower metabolisms than those who did not. Decreases in metabolic rate were associated with weight loss and regain in obese women (Jequier, 1990). Studies with rats also suggest that weight cycling increases the efficiency of feeding, that is, more weight is gained on less food (Brownell, 1986). Thus, a person who losses a large amount of weight and then rapidly regains it theoretically may have a lowered metabolic rate, making weight loss more difficult and increasing the likelihood of regaining weight during the next dieting attempt.

However, not all studies of weight cycling support these conclusions. Robison (1993) has shown that lowered metabolism with dieting to be only a temporary effect, and one that does not occur with diets containing at least 1,200 calories.

Some studies also suggest that weight cycling may increase death rate, particularly from heart disease (Lissner, 1991), whereas other studies fail to support such findings (Jeffrey, 1992). Repeated failure

to maintain weight loss may also contribute to the poor self-esteem experienced by many obese persons. Though still unclear, the possible negative effects of weight loss and regain deserve further study.

EFFECTIVE TREATMENT STRATEGIES

Obesity is not one condition but many conditions with varied causes. Oftentimes the exact cause of obesity is not well understood. The most effective treatment strategies for a particular obese person will depend on the cause of their obesity.

Treatment of obesity is complicated—there are no quick and easy fixes. Whereas weight loss is often possible though not easy, the real challenge is long-term weight control. Like treatment of many other chronic diseases, treatment of obesity requires long-term follow-up. A person with high blood pressure requires frequent monitoring and assessment of intervention strategies. An obese person also requires frequent monitoring and ongoing intervention and support. Even follow-up of six to twelve months may be too short. Follow-up lasting many years may be needed to ensure lifetime weight control (Bjorvell, 1992).

Effective obesity treatment programs must be individualized; different approaches work for different people. People who are involved in developing their own eating and exercise program are more likely to successfully lose weight and keep it off than people on a more rigid program (Kayman, 1990).

Effective treatment programs must also be comprehensive, involving a multi-disciplinary team of nurses, doctors, dietitians, exercise physiologists, psychologists, and other health professionals all working with the individual to achieve realistic weight goals (American Dietetic Association, 1989).

The focus of weight control efforts should be on improving health, not on improving cosmetic appearance. According to a recent National Institutes of Health Technology Assessment Conference (1992), weight loss treatments that "focus on approaches that can produce health benefits independently of weight loss may be the best way to improve the physical and psychological health of Americans seeking to lose weight."

At any one time, almost one-half of adult American women and one-quarter of American men are dieting to lose weight (Robison, 1993). Almost one-half of high-school age girls are dieting (Centers for Disease Control, 1991). These figures mean that the number of people dieting far exceeds the number of people who are actually obese.

Therefore many people, particularly young women, are dieting unnecessarily. Society is obsessed with thinness, putting intense pressure on women and increasingly on men to conform to unrealistic body weight ideals. These unrealistic ideals and cultural preoccupation with slimness are dangerous breeding grounds for development of eating disorders.

Goals for weight loss should be realistic, achievable, and emphasize gradual and permanent change in eating habits and exercise patterns for a lifetime of good health.

The most effective strategy for lifetime weight control is prevention. Nurses can help their patients reach and maintain weight loss goals by presenting objective information on causes and health effects of obesity, by promoting healthy eating and exercise behaviors for patients and their families, by monitoring weight fluctuations, and by recommending intervention at an early stage.

The next chapter examines some of the many causes of obesity. A greater understanding of the physiological, socio-cultural, and psychological factors that contribute to obesity will help nurses target the most appropriate interventions.

EXAM QUESTIONS

Chapter 1

Questions 1-8

1. Compared with the adult average, which of the following groups of Americans has a lower prevalence of obesity?

   a. white males
   b. black females
   c. minority populations
   d. older individuals

2. With increasing body mass index, death rate:

   a. remains unchanged
   b. increases in a J-shaped curve
   c. increases linearly
   d. decreases linearly

3. About what percentage of all Americans are overweight?

   a. less than 15%
   b. 15 to 20%
   c. 25 to 30%
   d. over 40%

4. Noticeable improvements in health and metabolic control have been documented with weight losses of:

   a. 40 percent of body weight
   b. 30 percent of body weight
   c. 20 percent of body weight
   d. 10 percent of body weight

5. Obesity increases risk of developing all of the following except:

   a. cardiovascular disease
   b. type I diabetes
   c. type II diabetes
   d. high blood pressure

6. Weight loss can cause:

   a. high blood pressure
   b. high blood cholesterol levels
   c. type II diabetes
   d. hair loss

7. The most challenging aspect of lifetime weight control is:

   a. maintaining weight loss over the long-term
   b. keeping up a regular exercise program
   c. decreasing caloric intake to 1,200 calories daily
   d. losing weight at a slow but steady rate

8. Effective obesity treatment programs must be:

   a. highly structured
   b. individualized
   c. family-oriented
   d. behavior-oriented

CHAPTER 2

WHY ARE SO MANY AMERICANS OVERWEIGHT?

CHAPTER OBJECTIVE

After completing this chapter, you will be able to explain some of the genetic, physiological, environmental, and psychological reasons why obesity is so prevalent in our society.

LEARNING OBJECTIVES

After studying this chapter, you will be able to:

1. Describe the importance of the number and type of fat cells.

2. Understand the role of the basal metabolic rate.

3. Determine the effects of gender on weight and weight loss.

4. Explain how patterns of overeating develop early in life and persist throughout adulthood.

5. List some behavioral differences between overweight adults and those of normal weight.

6. Explain how an altered sense of body image contributes to eating disorders.

INTRODUCTION

Most people in the United States live and move amid a world of abundant food. Unlike other cultures, where a large part of the day is spent gathering and preparing foods, Americans generally live and work within easy reach of grocery stores, convenience stores, fast-food outlets, and restaurants where food is available in large quantities with a minimum of effort.

In addition, our bodies, which were designed for maximum fuel-burning and fuel-storing efficiency, now run on "idle," even as we continue to eat much more efficiently than our ancestors ever did. For a few obese persons, an underlying metabolic defect worsens the problem.

This chapter analyzes the many physiological factors that help perpetuate excess weight gain and that may also work against the serious dieter. For most persons, excess weight may merely be a matter of too many calories and too little exercise; for others, however, complex genetic and metabolic components may be the cause.

Psychological factors that promote overeating are examined, including a barrage of food advertising, easy access to high-calorie foods, food attitudes, and internal forces that fuel overeating.

EVOLUTION OF OBESITY

Humans are among the fattest of all mammals — for example, the proportion of body fat to total body mass ranges from about 10 percent in the very lean to more than 35 percent in the obese (Brown and Konner, 1987). In other mammals, fat deposits offer protection and insulation from cold; in humans, fat serves as an energy reserve.

Anthropologists have made some interesting inroads into the causes of obesity. They note that for 95 to 99 percent of our history, humans lived exclusively as hunters and food gatherers, or foragers (Stuart, 1972). Oddly enough, some of the "contemporary food foragers" have characteristics in common with those ancestors. These contemporary food foragers live in small, socially flexible, semi-nomadic bands, experience slow population growth due to prolonged nursing and high childhood mortality, enjoy high-quality diets, spend proportionately little time directly involved in collecting food, and are generally healthier and better nourished than many contemporary Third World populations that depend upon agriculture for survival.

Although civilizations were able to progress once agriculture made year-round storage of food possible, an unfortunate byproduct of the change from forager to farmer was the opportunity for obesity to develop in people genetically predisposed to it.

According to some anthropologists, there are two reasons for the growth of obesity as a public health problem today: changes in eating habits of children and adults in developed countries, and changes in use of energy.

One dietary expert, Dr. George Christakis (1979) former director of the New York City Bureau of Nutrition, has another theory about the evolution of overnourished Americans. He notes that nutritionists developed broad-scale community education programs to increase consumption of foods rich in nutrients; unfortunately, they didn't educate children and their parents about the necessity of reducing other foodstuffs that are lacking in nutrition. This occurred at a time when eating became a recreational event, with the advent of snacking in front of the television, coffee breaks, cookouts, and dinner parties. At the same time, convenience foods became widely available.

Another factor also was at work — the impact of labor-saving devices, which changed normal energy needs. A simple example is the family car that replaced the walk to the school bus that replaced the bicycle that replaced the walk to school.

WHAT CAUSES OBESITY?

Obesity is not one disease but many diseases all characterized by excess adipose, or fat tissue. The underlying equation beneath all forms of obesity is *calories in versus calories out*. If energy intake is chronically greater than energy expenditure, obesity will result.

Obesity = energy intake > energy expenditure

Factors That Affect Energy Intake
- Appetite control
- Environmental influences
- Availability of food
- Diet composition

Factors That Affect Energy Expenditure
- Low metabolic rate
- Low level of physical activity
- Reduced thermogenesis (burning off calories as heat)

Factors that contribute to obesity include body metabolism, the environment we live and eat in, diseases of the endocrine glands, abnormalities in appetite regulation, abnormalities in fat (adipose) cell number and size, compulsive eating disorders, and effects of drugs (Willard, 1991). Nurses and other health professionals must consider the types and causes of obesity in designing appropriate treatment interventions.

GENETIC TENDENCIES

Recent studies yield increasing evidence that obesity is not merely the result of gluttony and sloth (Ravussin, 1992). Obese parents tend to have obese children. About 40 percent of children with one obese parent become obese; when both parents are obese, the risk of obesity rises to about 70 percent (Winick, 1985).

Animal studies have helped clarify questions about how much obesity is due to genetics and how much it is due to bad habits or lack of sufficient exercise. It is possible to breed strains of rats and mice that have a tendency to become obese; scientists do this by repeatedly breeding together the most obese animals. Logue et al. (1986) reported that genetically obese rats differ from normal rats in more ways than weight alone. Genetically obese rats consume the same amount of a single available sucrose solution as normal rats do. However, when genetically obese rats are given a choice between two sucrose solutions, the genetically obese rats have a lower preference for high concentrations of sucrose than normal rats do. This same difference is found in obese children and adults; in addition, the greater the difference, the greater the degree of obesity.

Thus, the relative aversion to high concentrations of sucrose by obese persons seems to support the idea that humans don't become obese by increasing the amount of sweet, highly caloric food in their diets.

To try to explain this phenomenon, special studies have been devised to examine the tendency to obesity in humans. Twins have provided a good model: In twin studies, the weights of identical and fraternal twins have been compared. Other studies have compared the weights of biological parents and their offspring and of adoptive parents and their adopted children. The outcome has usually been that weights tend to be more similar between identical twins than fraternal twins and more similar between parents and their offspring than adoptive parents and their adopted children (Bray, 1979; Price & Stunkard, 1989).

In a recent study of 4, 071 pairs of twins, Stunkard (1986) estimated that about 80 percent of obesity could be explained by genetics.

Many studies have shown that there is indeed a correlation between overweight in parents and in children. Obesity does run in families. In studies in Philadelphia, for example, Angel (1978) found that at least half of the children of obese-average parents were obese, and two-thirds of children of obese-obese parents were themselves obese. Eighty percent of the obese children had at least one fat parent. In another study (Stunkard and Stellar, 1984), when both parents were obese, their children had a 90 percent chance of being obese.

Stunkard (1984) examined genetic factors and obesity in 540 Danish adults who had been adopted as children. They found a strong relationship between the weight of the adoptees and the body mass index of the biologic parents, but no relation between the weight of the adoptees and their adoptive parents. They concluded that genetic tendencies have an important role in determining fatness in adults, whereas the family environment has a lesser impact.

The Pima Indians living in Arizona provided researchers with a model of genetic obesity (Ravussin, 1993). About 75 percent of the Pima Indians are obese, indicating that this form of obesity results from a genetically determined efficiecy of food use.

Mechanisms for the genetic tendency to become obese include a low metabolic rate, decreased ability to waste excess calories as heat (thermogenesis), and a set point for fat cell size. These and other contributors to obesity will be discussed in the next sections.

PHYSIOLOGICAL FACTORS

Low Metabolic Rate

Many overweight persons don't eat more than thin persons; in fact, many eat less. It is possible for an obese person to eat as few as 1,000 calories a day or even fewer, and yet stay at the same weight. In contrast, some thin persons can eat tremendous meals without gaining much weight (Simonson, 1983). The difference is that the fat person may be more fuel-efficient than the thinner one. As we mentioned before, the body becomes very efficient at storing incoming calories — this survival trait works to our disadvantage in times when food is plentiful.

Obese persons tend to have a lower metabolic rate than thinner persons, so they may need fewer calories to maintain their weight (Willard, 1991). Basal metabolic rate (BMR) is the amount of energy the body requires to maintain life when it is at digestive, physical, and emotional rest. The BMR is the rate at which stored energy is expended. This energy comes from burning stored fat and is measured by determining the amount of oxygen used to burn fat. The amount of oxygen consumed at rest is used as a measure of the basal energy requirements and is expressed as kilocalories per square meter of body surface per hour. The BMR is reported as the percentage of variation in the person above or below the normal number of kilocalories for a person of similar height, weight, and sex.

The BMR is measured in the following way: First, a patient who has fasted for at least eight hours lies comfortably awake in a darkened, quiet room while breathing oxygen from a machine, which measures the amount of oxygen used over a 15-minute period. The amount of oxygen used during that period reflects the quantity of energy used with the patient under basal conditions.

The test is always done with the patient in a fasting state because digestion and absorption of food also use energy, although the amount is small. However, even this slight amount would be enough to raise the basal metabolic rate. The BMR is also measured with indirect laboratory tests, such as thyroid function tests.

Most adults at rest require between 600 and 1,800 calories per 24 hours; this amount tends to correlate with the person's body size. Thus, the BMR is corrected for body size and is given as a certain percentage above or below normal, so that, theoretically at least, an NFL linebacker and a petite housewife should have the same range of basal metabolic rates. In reality, however, obese people have lower BMRs than thin persons (Winick, 1985).

The BMR depends on the mass of active cells, or the body cell mass. As Dr. Eric Jequier (1987) of the University of Lausanne in Switzerland has noted, the difficulty of any study that attempts to measure regulation of energy balance in humans is that it is very hard to measure small differences between energy intake and output. An adult man whose energy intake exceeded energy output by 5 percent each day for a whole year would gain about 125 kilocalories (kcal) per day, or 46,625 kcal in a year. If this man's energy intake surpassed his energy output by 5 percent a day for one year, he would gain about 7 kg a year.

In the past, measuring small differences in BMR after meals was difficult; old methods for measuring gas samples were uncomfortable for the patient and inaccurate because of air leaks. Now, however, it is much easier to measure BMR before and after meals using a ventilated hood system or a respiration chamber.

Total energy expenditure in a 24-hour period is made up of three components:

1. The basal metabolic rate,
2. The thermic effect of food (energy necessary to digest food), and
3. Energy cost of physical activity.

Of these three, basal metabolic rate makes up the greatest portion of energy expenditure.

Ravussin and Bogardus (1992) recently documented a large variability in basal metabolic rate among individuals independent of body weight, age, or sex. Some people may genetically have lower energy expenditures, making them at greater risk for obesity (Ravussin, 1993). In fact, prospective studies have shown that a low metabolic rate can predict future obesity in young adults (Ravussin, 1988) and infants (Roberts, 1988).

Although obese individuals may have lower metabolic rates, their total energy expenditure in 24 hours may actually be higher than that of thinner persons because of the greater energy cost maintaining and carrying around excess weight (Jequier, 1987). This implies that most obese persons must have a greater intake of daily energy than lean persons to maintain body weight and body composition.

Recent starvation, semistarvation, and rigorous or prolonged dieting can lower basal metabolic rate (Willard, 1991). Suppression of metabolic rate in such situations is the body's attempt to adapt to de-privation and to conserve energy. Thus dieting can become a contributor to obesity (Simonson, 1983).

Thermogenesis

Recently there has been increased interest in the role of thermogenesis and its effect on weight and the BMR. Thermogenesis refers to conditions that increase the BMR at rest, most importantly, dietary thermogenesis. Exposure to cold, ingestion of caffeine, and smoking are conditions that stimulate resting metabolic rate (Jequier, 1987).

Ingestion of food stimulates the metabolism and produces a demand for energy to meet the multiple activities of digestion, absorption, and transport of the nutrients. This overall stimulating effect of food is called its specific dynamic action, or more commonly, dietary thermogenesis. About 10 percent of the body's total energy needs for metabolism is attributed to metabolization of food. More metabolic work is involved to handle proteins, so that protein-rich foods stimulate basal metabolism more than any other nutrients.

Are there differences in the rate that men and women burn kilocalories? Traditional standards for calculating kilocalorie need would say yes; however, more modern research techniques (Simonson and Heilman, 1983) indicate there aren't sizable differences. In 1919, a study indicated that gender was a major factor in determining basal metabolic rate. Today, body surface area is used as a basis for calculating the resting metabolic rate (RMR). Because body surface area is generally less in women, resting metabolic rates are generally lower for women.

Women do have a lower resting metabolic rate. However, this is due to a smaller proportion of muscle mass to fat, not due to gender. (Some nutritionists and weight-loss experts maintain that men have a 6 to 7 percent higher BMR.)

The only factor that might seem to be gender-specific and that might influence the rate at which calories are burned is the menstrual cycle. Solomon, Kurzer, and Calloway (Simonson & Heilman, 1983) found that the BMRs of women studied during a 92-day period fell to their lowest points a week before ovulation, then rose gradually until the start of the next cycle. It is unclear how this affects weight loss, but some speculate that the lower kilocalorie needs during every menstrual cycle might pose a potential for chronic weight gain in some women.

Persons who skip meals regularly burn slightly less energy from dietary thermogenesis. Some evidence also indicates that skipping meals may decrease basal metabolic rate (Callaway, 1985).

Many individuals also have the ability to burn off a certain amount of excess calories as heat, a process called *adaptive thermogenesis*. Obese persons may have decreased adaptive thermogenesis, making them at risk for obesity (Lanzola, 1991; Poelman, 1986).

For some time, a unique fat cell has been of special interest to nutritionists and weight loss experts. This is the "brown fat cell," which derives its name from the cell's high concentration of brown pigment (Stuart & Davis, 1972). Brown fat, which makes up about 1 percent of body weight, is found at specific sites throughout the body. Brown fat cells have been found, for example, just above the kidneys, around the heart, along the aorta, and between the shoulder blades. Studies in laboratory animals have shown that this specialized brown adipose tissue has a primary function, burning off excess energy as heat, which it does at a much higher rate than ordinary fat cells. In obese animals, a defect interferes with this function. It isn't yet known how this defect may correlate with human obesity.

Diseases of the Endocrine System

Although rare, certain diseases are associated with obesity (Willard, 1991). Hypercortisolism, polycystic ovaries, hyperinsulinemia, some insulinomas,

and hypothyroidism can all promote obesity either through altered metabolism or appetite.

Use of inappropriate high doses of insulin in the treatment of diabetes also promotes obesity. Insulin triggers uptake of blood triglycerides into fat cells, favoring storage of excess calories as fat. In fact, the resistance to the action of insulin commonly seen in obesity and type II diabetes may be an adaptive response by the body to prevent additional weight gain (Eckel, 1992).

Adipose Cell Proliferation

The amount of body fat present at any one time is the amount by which acquired energy has exceeded energy use. Fatty, or adipose, tissue provides a very efficient way to store energy, and all animals tend to deposit fat into storage. As Dr. Grant Gwinup (1970) describes, fats, or hydrocarbons, are long chains of carbon atoms joined to hydrogen atoms. All forms of fat have two important characteristics: They do not mix with water and they give off large quantities of energy when they are burned.

Fat is an extremely efficient fuel — that is, this high-energy source has a relatively small volume and thus can be stored in a relatively small space. Gwinup also makes the interesting observation that all forms of life that move use fat or oil as the material in which their energy is stored. This is true for fish, animals, and birds, but also for seeds, which are rich in oil because they depend on the wind for mobility. In contrast, trees, bushes, and plants, which remain in one place, store energy as carbohydrates.

Although the human body is well able to use protein or carbohydrate as a fuel source, doing so would necessitate carrying about ten times the weight of either to gain the same amount of energy as is available from fat. One ounce of fat frees more than twice as much energy as an ounce of carbohydrate or an ounce of protein, and it can be stored almost free of water (a second characteristic of fat). Each ounce of protein or carbohydrate is stored with 3 or 4 ounces of water (Gwinup, 1970).

Our body cells also store fat in a very efficient manner. Each cell, which is about 1/100,000th-inch in diameter, is enclosed in a thin, flexible membrane that adheres to the membranes of surrounding cells. Fat is stored in connective tissue cells, which have the ability to store tremendous amounts of fat. Any connective tissue cell can become a fat cell merely by filling itself with fat. When it becomes a fat cell, it swells, stretching the cell membrane so that it is no longer ovoid and pointed on each end, but now becomes round and distended, like a beach ball. It can expand to many times its original size; in addition, the fat in the cell pushes the nucleus out to the edge of the cell. The cell is supplied with a small blood vessel, which acts as a conduit for taking up fats and releasing them back into the bloodstream; each cell is also supplied with tiny nerve fibers.

Our body is a tremendously efficient energy storage unit; we have millions of connective tissue cells that can easily become fat cells. Thus, our bodies have a nearly unlimited ability to store up fat. It is as if, as Gwinup (1970) says, a car's gas tank could swell from a capacity of 1 gallon to 1,000 gallons, depending upon the availability of gasoline.

When we eat a meal, the following mechanisms go into action: The portion that is carbohydrate is disposed of. A small amount is burned by the body to provide energy, a small amount is stored in the liver as an emergency source of carbohydrate, and most is changed to fat and stored in the fat cells.

Part of the protein from the meal is used to repair muscle breakdown that has occurred since protein was last eaten, but the amount of protein beyond this amount is quickly changed to carbohydrate by the liver. Nitrogen is removed and excreted via the urine. The carbohydrate that is produced is taken to the fat cells, where it is converted to fat.

A small amount of the fat that has been consumed at this meal is burned to take care of immediate energy needs, but most is carried to the fat cells, where it is stored as a reserve energy source.

Thus whether you eat fat, carbohydrate, or protein, the same amount of body fat will be produced. A person can become obese from too much protein as well as from too much carbohydrates, if the intake of energy exceeds the energy use (Gwinup, 1970).

Between meals, the need for energy is communicated through the minute nerve cells that connect with each fat cell; these cells transmit the message that more energy or fat is needed, and stored fat is converted into energy until more food is consumed. Thus, the cell's ability to store fats has enabled man to lead a life that is free of continued consumption of food in order to supply energy needs.

Recently, much attention has turned to the number and size of fat cells, and their influence on weight. A person may have a normal number of fat cells that are swelled with an excess of fat, while another may have too many fat cells. We are all born with our own genetic makeup of fat cells. Some of us are born with more fat cells.

In a series of studies (Bray, 1985) first done at Rockefeller University, New York City, and later verified by studies at other universities in the United States and abroad, it was shown that weight reduction is always accompanied by a shrinkage in fat-cell size, but not by a reduction of fat cell numbers.

Dr. Myron Winick (1985), nutritionist and weight control expert at Columbia University, New York City, described what happens when a person with too many fat cells diets down to his or her ideal weight:

> Suppose a person had twice as many fat
> cells as normal and that each cell contained
> just the right amount of fat. Such a person
> would be quite obese, since his or her body

would contain twice as much total fat as it should. In order for that individual to achieve normal weight, half of the fat from each cell would have to be burned. Thus, the fat cells would shrink to half their normal size. If now we examined the fatty tissue of this person, who has painfully dieted down to ideal weight, it would appear more abnormal than when he or she was obese. There would be too many cells, which are now too small as well. The body somehow senses this double abnormality and struggles to rectify the situation by trying to fill those 'depleted' fat cells with more fat. For this reason, it is extremely difficult for a person whose obesity is primarily due to too many fat cells to lose weight, and it is even more difficult for that person to maintain the weight loss for a long time.

In contrast, for the person with a normal number of fat cells each containing twice as much fat as it should, weight is easier to lose and weight loss is easier to maintain. As this person loses weight, the fat cells shrink and when an ideal weight is attained, the fat cells are of normal size. Everything is at the proper level and thus is much easier to maintain.

How does a person develop an abnormal number of fat cells? Usually the total number of fat cells is reached by early adolescence. Thereafter fat cells usually increase in size only, not in number.

However, fat cells seem to have an upper limit as to how far they can stretch (Willard, 1992). Fat cells in people who are normal weight are about $0.5\mu g$ in diameter. With weight loss, fat cells decrease to about $0.4\mu g$. In most types of obesity, fat cells can increase to 0.7 to $1.0\mu g$, but they rarely exceed $1.5\mu g$. At this massively obese point, cells have reached their maximum size, and the formation of new fat cells is triggered again. Once more fat cells

have been made, they are permanent, making long-term weight loss difficult for severely obese individuals.

Appetite Regulation

In most people, physiological hunger is carefully regulated by a series of checks and balances controlled by the hypothalamus gland (Blundell, 1990). The hypothalamus senses changes in physical activity and food intake and sends out signals in a very accurate fashion when more food is needed. Interestingly, however, people who are very sedentary may have a faulty check and balance system. Researchers have shown that a low activity level is associated with inappropriately high levels of food intake in both animals and humans (Brownell, 1980).

Though very rare, certain diseases of the hypothalamus, such as Prader-Willi syndrome, can cause voracious appetite and lead to obesity.

Set Point

Obesity is often regarded as a failure of regulation, or lack of balance of intake and expenditure of energy. Biological scientists have found the *set-point principle* useful for describing the systems that regulate such physiologic variables as body temperature and blood pressure. The set-point theory of weight (Keesey, 1988) is the particular value of a regulated variable at which the system is in balance or stasis.

Currently, it is believed that each person is programmed to have a certain degree of fatness or a body weight at which he or she tends to remain, or has a "set point" for weight. Like a thermostat, the set point keeps weight within a relatively narrow range; sometimes it spontaneously jumps, adding a few pounds every five years or so. It is believed that a regulatory mechanism in the brain senses and adjusts both our appetite and our energy use. Thus, when the degree of fat content falls below its programmed amount, and you start to lose weight, you unconsciously desire more food; when you return to your set point, appetite slackens, and you unconsciously begin eating less.

Animal studies have been very helpful for demonstrating the set point and its effects on weight gain and loss. Three types of rodent models have provided some information on set point: the Zucker "fatty" rat, which has genetically transmitted obesity, dietary obesity, and hypothalamic obesity. In the Zucker rat, obesity is inherited as a single recessive gene. Early in the development of obesity, both over-consumption of calories and enhanced energy efficiency contribute to the obesity. The increasingly efficient use of energy can be traced to a reduced rate of resting metabolism, which scientists can detect several days after birth. When the rat becomes an obese adult, it defends its body weight by exercising the correct control over energy intake and energy expenditure. Even if its diet is made unpalatable by the addition of quinine, the rat will eat enough of it to maintain its high body weight. It also lowers its resting metabolism if its weight is reduced from its normally high limits (Keesey, 1988).

A particular type of diet can also induce obesity in rats. When laboratory rats are offered certain very palatable diets or a selection of "junk" foods, their natural resistance to weight gain is overcome and they become obese (Sclafani and Springer, 1985). If such rats are kept on a high-fat diet for six months, they are no longer hypermetabolic; instead, the number of fat cells increases and resting heat production is reduced to a level that is normal for that particular amount of body weight. If their weight declines, they effectively reduce energy use; then, when there is only mild calorie restriction, their resting metabolic rate falls much lower than that of normal-weight rats. Rats who have had bilateral destruction of their hypothalamus eat two to three times normal amounts, which leads to a massive weight gain, all as fat. Unlike rats with genetic and dietary causes for obesity, rats with hypothalamic obesity do not defend their obesity; that is, they fail to adjust intake when weight is challenged, and

when unpalatable food is present weight declines to normal or lower-than-normal levels (Keesey, 1988).

Many obese persons seem to regulate their weight in a normal fashion, and seem to need about the same or slightly more calories for maintaining daily weight as normal-weight persons do.

The basal metabolic rate may also change to suit the circumstances. It automatically slows down to conserve energy and speeds up to burn it, more or less keeping weight stable (Keesey, 1988). Thus, theoretically at least, the set point is a physiological control center that keeps weight at a constant level. For some persons, obesity seems to be regulated. These persons have energy-conserving metabolic adaptations that resist weight change and probably lessen their chances of losing significant amounts of weight or keeping off weight lost through dieting. In order for these people to keep weight off, they must make a lifelong commitment to a daily intake of calories that probably won't satisfy their hunger and that may be less than that consumed by normal-weight persons.

Experts disagree whether a set point for body weight exists. If it does exist, it may be possible to change a person's set point by adjusting diet and increasing physical activity levels (Simonson, 1983).

Pharmacological Effects

Some medications can promote weight gain (Willard, 1992) by increasing appetite or changing metabolism. Such medications include tricyclic antidepressants, phenothiazines, oral contraceptives, and glucocorticoids.

Smoking cigarettes may increase metabolic rate (Perkins, 1989), so when a persons stops smoking weight gain may result. Modest weight gain, however, is still preferable to the unhealthy consequences of smoking. Changes in appetite control may also trigger weight gain after smoking cessation.

Racial and Gender Differences

Average body weight differs with race and gender. Overweight increases with age in both sexes. Minority populations have a higher prevalence of obesity than white men and women. Obesity in black women is more common in all age groups than in white women. Among black men, however, this racial difference is only present between the ages of 35 and 54. Although obesity is also more prevalent among people with lower incomes, the racial differences in obesity rate persist even when controlling for socioeconomic status.

Generally, it is physiologically easier for men to stay thin because their bodies contain more muscle tissue and less fatty tissue than women's bodies. While men may weigh more than women, less of their weight is fat (Simonson, 1983).

Obesity in women is more likely to develop at certain periods of life: the first three years of life, during adolescence, and the third trimester of pregnancy. Women usually gain weight after age 20, during or after pregnancy, and during menopause. Women also start adding fatty tissue during the teenage years because of the release of estrogen. In contrast, men usually lose weight during their teenage years, largely due to the effects of testosterone. Testosterone promotes development of muscle tissue.

Because men have more muscle tissue than women, they burn calories more quickly than women do. Thus, men need almost twice as many calories to maintain the same weight. Men are almost always taller and heavier because of a larger skeleton, so they require more energy for activity. Thus, men can lose weight at nearly twice the rate as women even though they are eating exactly the same number of calories. The average active man loses weight even though he may be taking in as many as 2,000 to 2,200 calories a day, while the average woman must cut calories to the 1,000 to 1,200 calorie per day level to lose weight.

Women's bodies are made up of a much higher percentage of fat. Some scientists note that this is a superior survival element, but not too many women are exposed to sub-zero temperatures or starvation, which would make this trait come in handy! A normal college-aged man's body is made up of about 15 percent fat. A woman of the same age, 20 years old, for example, is about 25 percent fat, half of which is stored right under the skin — the advanced survival element. By the time she reaches 55 years of age, the proportion of body fat will rise to about 38 percent (Simonson, 1983).

Women's fat also accumulates in the body in a different pattern than men's. Women's fat usually accumulates below the waist, and weight gain tends to occur all over the body. In contrast, men's fat is distributed far more evenly throughout the body and when they gain weight, it tends to be deposited more evenly throughout the back, midsection, necks, and just over the navel.

Men and women also tend to have different weight gain patterns. For example, tall men (those taller than 5'8") reach peak weights between 35 and 45 years of age; shorter men take longer to reach peak weights. These men keep adding weight until they are between 45 and 55 years of age before their weight begins leveling off.

Women begin adding weight in their teens, and continue to gain weight until they are 55 to 64 years old. Weight jumps up for them with each pregnancy and again at menopause.

Women also have greater weight fluctuations than men because of their ever-changing hormonal levels throughout the menstrual cycle. As progesterone levels rise in relation to the amount of estrogen available and circulating throughout the body just before menstruation occurs, women tend to retain water in their tissues. For women who do not produce enough estrogen to counterbalance the progesterone, it is common to gain 5 to 6 or more pounds right before menstruation.

Premenstrual women crave extra amounts of sweet or salty foods; chocolate in any form seems to be a particular favorite. When researchers (Simonson, 1983) studied this common phenomenon, they found that it usually peaks on the second day of the menstrual period. Overweight women seem to have much greater cravings for these types of foods than normal-weight women do; the heavier the woman, the more intense the desire for such foods becomes.

There may be a reasonable physiologic explanation for this: One theory (Stunkard, 1980) holds that women have a shortage of progesterone or a drop in the level of beta endorphins, endogenous brain polypeptides that raise the pain threshold during menstruation. The fall in beta endorphins causes a reduction in the serotonin supply. Serotonin acts as a mood elevator and appetite suppressor. Others believe (Simonson, 1983) that low levels of blood sugar just before the menstrual period lead to the urge to binge on sweet and salty foods.

Women also have a tendency to gain weight after the menopause; no one yet has found out why this occurs. The shape of the body also changes at this time. Fat is lost around the hips, thighs, and breasts, and is gained in the waistline, rib cage area, and back.

Why do men develop so-called "beer bellies" more often than women? Often, it isn't just the natural result of gaining weight, since some men develop protruding abdomens even when they haven't gained many pounds. The true cause is usually lax abdominal muscles that then add layers of fat over the muscle. After eating fewer calories and exercising more, they find that the area firms up again.

Dr. Simonson (1983) adds a final physiologic note about obese people that is worth contemplating. In her book, *The Complete University Medical Diet*, she

writes, "Very few, very old people are truly obese. That's because fat people die younger."

ENVIRONMENTAL INFLUENCES

Effects of Prolonged Dieting

Going on a series of drastic diets that cause constant weight loss and gain may impair the metabolic process, making it harder to return to a normal weight and stay there. Dieting can then become the major cause of overweight and obesity (Simonson, 1983).

According to Dr. Simonson (1983), increased fuel efficiency can also result from being overweight. Persistent overweight, rapid changes in weight, and stringent dieting can change the body's biochemistry, actually slowing down the metabolism, so that a person needs fewer calories per day to keep her overweight than she did to make her overweight in the first place.

As a person acquires more fatty tissue, which can be maintained at a lower energy cost than muscle tissue, the metabolism slows down so that less energy is expended. The body adjusts, becoming a more efficient machine; that is, it uses less fuel to maintain its needs. When a person stops a very low-calorie diet, the body remains at the lower metabolic rate for weeks or even months. With each diet, or each attempt to diet, the energy-saving slowdown of the metabolism is enhanced. It thus becomes increasingly difficult to take off pounds. At Rockefeller University, an endocrinological study center, researchers (Bray, 1985) have found that many obese persons can maintain their weight using a third to a half as many calories as persons of normal weight. Thus, a normal-weight person may need 2,000 calories a day to maintain body weight, while a 350-

pound person needs only 1,200 or fewer to maintain his weight.

Cultural and Family Environment

The family environment has a lot to do with habitual overeating. When too much food is the norm and where the quantity and the quality of the food are overemphasized by constant conversation about it, it's common for family members to consistently overeat. The types of foods are, of course, also important — it does make a difference if your staple foods are heavy, fried foods, or salads and fresh fruits, with lean meats.

Purposeful, or cortical overeating, can be a reflex by a child to silence a mother who is nagging him to eat. Illness may be another cause of purposeful overeating. In some cases, a high-calorie, high-protein diet is prescribed to help combat loss of vital tissue after a serious operation or an injury, but once the tissue destruction has stopped and the lost tissue is restored, there is no need to continue overfeeding. Mostly, purposeful overfeeding is due to ig-

norance. It is a misconception that eating beyond energy needs or growth requirements will give a person added strength. All it really does is lead to fat.

Cultural factors also promote obesity. Eating is a social and recreational activity. The job environment often encourages overeating.

Television viewing may also promote obesity. In teenagers, the number of hours spent watching television correlates with prevalence of obesity in an almost linear fashion (Figure 2.1). It is not clear whether excessive television watching causes obesity, or whether the reverse is true.

Socioeconomic Status

Obesity is more common among people with lower incomes, particularly among women. Kahn and colleagues studied 514 black women and 2,770 white women ages 25 to 44 years old over a 10-year interval to determine socioeconomic factors that might predict weight gain (Kahn, 1991). Women most at

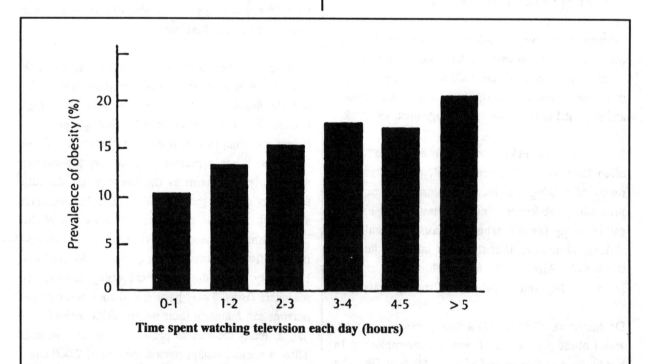

Figure 2.1 Television viewing correlated with prevalence of obesity.
Source: Willard, M.D. (June, 1991). Obesity: Types and Treatments. *American Family Physician* 43, 2099–108. Reprinted with permission by the American Academy of Family Physicians.

risk for gaining weight were those without a college education, those who married, and those with very low family incomes. Being a female from a minority population with a low socioeconomic status is considered a triple threat for obesity development (Bowen, 1991).

Sherry and colleagues (1992) studied the effect of socioeconomic status on obesity in children. Contrary to findings in adults, obesity was 50 percent more common in children from higher incomes than from lower incomes, although obesity was the most prevalent growth problem observed in both groups of children.

PSYCHOLOGICAL FACTORS

Food and Attitudes

Food is one of the most powerful commodities in our lives, one that directly affects our bodies and our behavior. Our attitudes about food are an often overlooked part of our heritage. Ethnic, socioeconomic, and environmental factors also influence the type and amount of food we like to eat.

Our society uses food for many reasons besides satisfying hunger. For example, food can be used as a reward for accomplishment, as means of celebrating special occasions, or as a way to express happiness and vitality. Nearly every type of celebration is accompanied by eating and drinking. Despite our culture's strong emphasis on thinness, extravagant overeating is the accepted method of celebrating any occasion, from weddings and birthdays to Christmas and New Year's Day.

Food can also provide a temporary sense of control over the physical world that surrounds us. In fact, food may at times seem to be the only thing that we can completely control. Food can replace feelings of emptiness, and may compensate for professional or personal failures or for lack of gratification. An individual can fight back against loneliness and sexual inadequacy with food, or it may help one put aside feelings of depression. In contrast, other people may use food as a target, to get rid of hostility, anger, fear, resentfulness, frustration, or as a release for otherwise unacceptable emotions.

Extra weight can become a barrier between ourselves and our responsibilities. Excess weight may act like a fortress, keeping away unwanted attention or sexuality. Extra weight can be a symbol of power, making a person feel more substantial, someone to be reckoned with and not ignored. Excess weight can also provide a way to avoid competing in a business setting.

Being markedly overweight may also be the result of a need for perfection. Dr. Simonson (1983) has found this pattern most often in women who feel they must have nearly complete control over their destinies. The slightest hint that they don't have complete control leads to a "food attack."

Dr. Simonson provides several psychological insights into obesity in her book, *The Complete University Medical Diet*:

1. The earlier the pattern of overeating begins, the earlier you lose your ability to know when and if you are physically hungry. At this point, it becomes more difficult to discriminate between hunger and anxiety.

2. The person who overuses food in an attempt to relieve anxiety tends to be one who is particularly sensitive to physical and emotional pain. Compared with normal controls, overweight people as a group show more concern about their bodies and their emotional equilibrium and less tolerance for discomfort.

3. Most seriously overweight people like to eat in the easiest way possible and want their food readily available.

In one study (Simonson, 1983), for example, researchers studied obese and thin persons by offering subjects nuts that were either wrapped in foil or unwrapped and loose. Thin subjects ate just as many nuts that were wrapped in foil as nuts that were unwrapped. In contrast, obese subjects ate many more unwrapped nuts, presumably because they were easier to get to.

When Dr. Simonson repeated this experiment at Johns Hopkins, using finger foods and foods that required a knife and a fork, the thin control subjects ate much smaller portions of both types of food than the obese group and did not differentiate between the types of food. Heavy subjects consumed three times as much finger foods as foods that required the use of a knife and fork.

4. Overweight persons are particularly sensitive to food-related environments. Dr. Simonson notes that this may help explain why many persons lose large amounts of weight while in the controlled setting of a hospital, a weight-loss camp, or health spa but quickly revert to their former shapes and sizes as soon as they are back in their home environment. This is especially true for children who are sent away to "fat camps."

5. It has also been learned that once a person who has been consistently obese starts eating, it usually takes him longer to feel satisfied and to stop eating than it does a normal person. Thus, even if he doesn't eat more often than normal, he manages to eat more before his brain receives the signal that hunger has been satisfied.

Psychological Disturbances

Some researchers (Mendelson & White, 1982) feel that obesity is caused by varying degrees of psychological disturbances. For them, there is a virtual spectrum of overweight patients, ranging from those with slight problems with food to those who are obsessed with food. At one end of the spectrum are people who are emotionally stable but overweight. These people may overeat during times of stress, for example. A second point on the spectrum involves people who eat to defend themselves against emotional tension, and for whom obesity is not really a major problem. Another group may overeat almost constantly as a means of warding off emotional upheavals. At the far end of the spectrum are severely disturbed people with a major obesity problem, who seem to be primarily preoccupied with finding and consuming food.

Personality Defects

Dr. Bruch (1978) is well known for her work with patients who have eating disorders, particularly anorexic patients. She has written that obesity is the consequence of personality defects in which body size becomes the expression of an underlying psychological conflict. The roots of the problem seem to lie in early life experiences.

Other scientists (Stunkard, 1980; Stuart, 1972) believe obesity develops as a result of problems during the "anal" period of childhood development, which is thought to be the point at which a young child seeks to establish his independence, while the parents try to bring the child's bowel and bladder habits under control. The conflicts during toilet training, when the child attempts to become independent while his parents seek to control him, theoretically lead to the character structure of an adult fixated at or preoccupied with the anal state. Such persons become concerned with orderliness, or compulsiveness, autonomy, and/or defenses against heterosexuality. Psychologists assert that overeating is a compulsive habit in which the person manifests his defiance of those who would control his eating while at the same time protecting himself from heterosexual experiences by virtue of the invulnerability or unattractiveness of excess weight.

Some people love to eat not because they need to satisfy a deep-seated emotional need, but because they can't deny themselves anything they really want, including the pleasure of eating. Some were trained from early on to be "good children," which meant eating heartily and cleaning every scrap from their plates. In adulthood, many overeaters still feel that limiting their intake of food is a betrayal of their parents and family traditions, even if their parents are no longer around to remind them to eat everything on their plates (Stuart, 1972).

Dr. Bruch (1979) has also theorized that one of the mechanisms by which parents inadvertently induce their children to become obese is through inappropriate use of food in response to varying emotional stress signals by the child, and conversely a failure to respond with food when the child becomes hungry. Because of this, food can become an inappropriate response to almost any strong emotion; thus, we may learn highly inappropriate responses and develop inappropriate food habits. Thus, eating disturbances — which can include anorexia as well as obesity — are often the result of pathogenic interaction between the individual and key figures in his environment.

Dr. Bruch (1979) has found certain patterns among parents and children that may be precursors to obesity. She has written:

> The early feeding histories of many fat and anorexic patients have been reconstructed with great detail. Often they are conspicuous by their blandness. The parents feel that there is nothing to report: the child never gave any trouble, ate exactly what was put before him; the mother was the envy of her friends and neighbors because her child did not fuss about food, nor was he negativ-

istic during the classic "period of resistance." This goodness was reported for other areas, too, like cleanliness, no rough play or destructive behavior, and no disobedience or back talking. Several mothers . . . would report with pride how they always "anticipated" their child's needs, never permitting him to "feel hungry."

Some specialists (Stunkard, 1980) in personality development have theorized that there is an unconscious association to the meaning of food itself, ranging from a substitute for motherly love to a belief that food is a symbol of the mother's breast, for example, or the father's phallus. Another group has tried to draw a link between overeating and the symbolic act of oral intake and digestion. Some of these theories can become very drawn out and too complex to be discussed here.

Yet another group (Stuart, 1979) believes that overeating represents a wide variety of behaviors, ranging from self-indulgence to a method of self-punishment. Using this theory, it may be possible to understand why some people resist losing weight. Conrad was among the psychologists who attributed resistance to dieting to an unwillingness by the obese person to lessen the usefulness of oral mechanisms as a way to solve emotional problems, to rebelliousness and an interest in preserving independence, to guilt when going off diets, to difficulty in being self-assertive when problem foods are encountered, to hesitance in giving up eating as a primary source of pleasure, and to a lack of motivation associated with a fear of failure.

The main problem with these theories is that researchers (Stuart, 1978) haven't yet found a way to prove them with controlled studies. Others (Stunkard, 1980) have found that it isn't possible to define psychological characteristics of obese patients that will consistently distinguish them from non-obese patients. This will be important to you in your efforts to work with obese and seriously overweight patients. It underscores the importance of individualizing your approach to persons with weight problems.

Eating Behaviors

Many have tried to find behavioral differences between obese persons and those of normal weight. Two scientists, Spitzer and Rodin (1975), examined the medical literature and found several things:

1. Obese people are more likely than normal-weight people to eat large amounts of palatable foods.

2. People who are obese are less likely to slow their rate of eating during the course of a meal than are normal-weight people.

3. During the course of an entire meal, there is no difference in the eating rates of obese and normal-weight people.

Many studies have been done to try to prove that food cues act as triggers for hunger among obese persons. Nisbett and his co-workers (Simonson, 1983) did find that obese persons were more subject to the influence of food cues than non-obese persons. They set up the following experiment to study the use of food cues.

Obese and non-obese subjects were deceived into believing they were participating in a study of psychophysiological responses. After a short period of interacting with meaningless but impressive procedures, the subjects were led into a second room, where they were asked to fill out questionnaires that they had been led to believe were related to the psychophysiological session.

In the room they found either one or three roast beef sandwiches and a bottle of a soft drink. They were told that since they would miss lunch because of the time involved in filling out the questionnaires, they were entitled to eat as many sandwiches

as they wanted, and were able to take more sandwiches out of the refrigerator at will.

The obese subjects did eat more sandwiches than the non-obese when three sandwiches were in sight; however, when only one sandwich was in view, they ate less than the normal subjects.

This study demonstrated that food cues — in this case the sandwiches — often have a powerful impact on obese people. They ate because the food was there, following visual cues, not because of any hunger cues.

To examine whether an obese person's state of mind has an impact upon overeating, three researchers, Schachter, Goldman, and Gordon (Stuart, 1972) devised an experiment among obese and non-obese subjects using a high degree of fear (severe electrical shocks) and low degree of fear (mild electrical shocks). Subjects were asked not to eat before the experiment, and then were shown a large console of electrical equipment. One group was told that they would be exposed to a severe shock to test the interaction between stimulation and taste; the second group was told that they might at most feel a slight tingle. Half of the subjects were offered a roast beef sandwich and a glass of water; the other half were offered no food or drink. Both groups were asked to taste and rate crackers during a 15-minute period before the shock. Shock wasn't ever used in either group.

The researchers found that whereas one group of normal-weight people (low fear, deprivation group) ate almost twice the number of crackers as those in the three other groups, obese persons ate slightly but not significantly more crackers during the time of high fear. The obese subjects also reported having more fear than the normal-weight persons. These results refuted the common idea that eating is more likely to reduce discomfort produced by fear in obese persons than in normal-weight persons.

In another study (Stuart, 1972), the impact of understimulation, or boredom, upon overeating was tested using several different types of "test foods." False feedback from the questioner showed that obese subjects ate more if they felt rejected by the interviewer, while normal subjects weren't affected. The conclusion was that obese subjects in the rejection condition reported a sharp decrease in boredom after eating, while normal subjects reported increased boredom after eating.

Internal versus External Control

In the late 1960s, Schachter (1971) and his colleagues developed the hypothesis that people of normal weight eat in response to internal physiological cues, especially hunger, whereas obese people eat because of external cues in their immediate environment. Thus, instead of feeling hungry and then eating as a response, obese persons eat in response to the time of day, the sight and nearness and accessibility of food, or the sight of other people eating. To test this theory, Schachter devised a study in which he changed the clocks in the study room to reflect a later time, closer to dinner time. The obese persons in the study ate twice as many snack crackers when they thought it was 6 p.m. than when they thought it was 5:20 p.m. Normal-weight persons acted in a very different way: They ate less, as if they were "saving" themselves for dinner.

Many overweight persons suffer from psychological problems that are directly related to obesity. One important problem is self-belittlement about body image.

The next chapter examines the serious effects obesity has on many of the body's systems. Obesity can dramatically shorten life span.

EXAM QUESTIONS

Chapter 2

Questions 9-18

9. Which factor does not affect energy intake?

    a. diet composition
    b. adaptive thermogenesis
    c. availability of food
    d. environmental influences

10. An abnormal number of fat cells usually develop at what age?

    a. during adulthood
    b. from fetal life through early adolescence
    c. in old age
    d. in late adolescence

11. The change from a nation of hunters to an agricultural society led to:

    a. no noticeable changes in average weights
    b. depletion of food stores
    c. opportunity for obesity to develop
    d. greater protein intake

12. Compared with normal-weight individuals, most obese persons eat:

    a. about 1,000 more calories daily
    b. about 500 more calories daily
    c. slightly more calories daily
    d. about the same or fewer calories daily

13. Which of the following conditions may cause obesity?

    a. hypertension
    b. atherosclerosis
    c. hyperlipidemia
    d. hypercortisolism

14. Which of the following is not a part of total energy expenditure in a 24-hour period?

    a. energy cost of adaptive thermogenesis
    b. basal metabolic rate
    c. thermic effect of food
    d. energy cost of physical activity

15. One of the main reasons it is easy to lose weight in a controlled setting such as a spa or hospital is:

    a. less food is served there
    b. overweight persons are especially susceptible to food-related environments
    c. motivation is higher
    d. institutionalized food is low in calories and fat

16. It is usually easier for men to lose weight than women because:

    a. they have better control over food intake
    b. they spend more time exercising
    c. they have greater fuel efficiency
    d. they have higher body muscle content

17. Compared with normal-weight individuals, obese individuals are more responsive to which type of food cues?

    a. taste
    b. appetite
    c. genetic
    d. visual

18. Most cases of obesity are the result of:

    a. genetic differences
    b. a chronic imbalance between intake and expenditure of energy
    c. a diet high in carbohydrates
    d. a low metabolic rate

CHAPTER 3

THE HIGH COST OF OBESITY

CHAPTER OBJECTIVE

After reading this chapter, you will be able to identify the many ways that obesity and marked overweight contribute to serious medical problems and recognize how obesity can affect societal attitudes and body image.

LEARNING OBJECTIVES

After studying this chapter, you will be able to:

1. Discuss some of the findings from several prospective studies, including the Framingham study, the American Cancer Society study, the Norwegian study, and the Nurses' Health Study.

2. Explain factors that increase the risk of atherosclerosis.

3. Describe how overweight affects cardiovascular disease, hyperlipidemia, hypertension, glucose intolerance, cancer, and other diseases.

INTRODUCTION

Not withstanding the magnitude of the billion-dollar diet industry, medical costs resulting from death and disease attributable to obesity are far greater. "Overweight is risking fate," says Dr. George A. Bray (1979), a leading authority on obesity and weight control. Being overweight escalates the risk of developing serious health problems such as coronary atherosclerosis, diabetes, cancer, hypertension, and hyperlipidemia.

This chapter scrutinizes the long-term effects of excess weight on society, self-perception of the body, and on life expectancy.

SOCIETAL ATTITUDES AND DISCRIMINATION

America's contempt for the obese and its preoccupation with thinness are evident everywhere. Researchers such as Dr. Thomas Waddell and Dr. Albert Stunkard (1980) of the University of Pennsylvania have found concrete evidence of the powerful prejudice against the obese that cuts across age, sex, race, and socioeconomic status.

Wadden and Stunkard (1986) note:

> Children as young as six years describe silhouettes of an obese child as "lazy," "dirty," "stupid," "ugly," "cheats," and "liars." When shown black and white drawings of a normal weight child, an obese child, and children with various handicaps, including missing hands and facial disfigurement, children and adults rated the obese child as the least likable. Not only is this prejudice relatively uniform among blacks and whites and persons from rural and urban settings, it is also, sadly, seen among obese persons themselves.

In a study of black and white males and females with college and high school educations, all groups, including overweight persons themselves, rated overweight children as least likable. When they were asked to label overweight persons with a wide choice of descriptive phrases, the obese were more likely to be described in less flattering terms. In a study of obese and normal-weight persons, test subjects were less likely to comply with requests from obese people than people of normal weight.

Discrimination against the obese can be found in lower acceptance rates into prestigious colleges for obese high school students compared with normal-weight students, despite identical high school performance and academic qualifications or application rates to colleges.

Obese persons may also encounter discrimination when they seek jobs and while on the job. Employers may rate overweight people as less desirable than normal-weight individuals, even when they think the two groups have the same abilities.

The stigma attached to being overweight can take a toll on the emotional health of some obese people. The negative attitude toward overweight is particularly strong toward women. The pressure, especially for women, to be slim is reflected all around us, particularly in advertising. Heavy persons are often perceived as less intelligent, or as negative or comical characters.

Many obese people describe themselves just as harshly as non-obese critics do. They note that they are unhappy with themselves and as a result have low self-esteem. In children, there seems to be some relationship between body-esteem and self-esteem (Gilbert, 1975). This appears to be true for obese as well as thin children, and often results in self-belittlement about body image. The way a person sees himself or herself is believed to have a powerful influence over the way in which he or she deals with food.

Negative attitudes toward obese people also exist within the nursing profession itself. In a study of female university students in a junior nursing class, Stein (1987) noted lower self-concept among obese students as compared to non-obese students. Another study evaluated affect neutrality of nurses toward normal-weight and over-weight patients (Peternelji-Taylor, 1989). Questionnaire analysis demonstrated that obese patients were evaluated more negatively than normal weight patients.

DISTORTED BODY IMAGE

Emotionally healthy obese persons have no body-image disturbances. However, certain obese people have serious problems with body image. Characteristically, they view themselves as grotesque and loathsome, and believe that other persons view them with hostility and contempt. Such persons are completely preoccupied with their obesity and related feelings of self-loathing; this is an internalization of parental and peer criticism, which persists when such criticism is no longer present.

This problem is seen most often in young middle- and upper-class women, groups in which obesity is less common and for whom sanctions are stronger. The disturbance is usually limited to persons who have been obese since childhood, who have a generalized neurotic disorder, and whose parents and friends have scolded them for being overweight (Stuart, 1979).

OBESITY AND MORTALITY

Life insurance statistics clearly show that excess weight is linked with increased mortality. Data from the Build Study of 1979 (American Society of Actuaries and Association of Life Insurance Medical Directors of America, 1980) show that the lowest mortality rates are in those individuals slightly under established weight for height in life insurance tables. Weights above or below this norm are associated with increased mortality. Others have found well-defined evidence about the effects of gross obesity on life expectancy. In one study, 200 morbidly obese men, whose average weight was 143.5 kg (315.7 lb) were interviewed when they were admitted into a weight control program. These men were followed for an average of 5 years. Their ages ranged from 23 to 70 years, with a mean of 42.7 years.

The mortality of this group was higher at every age when compared with the mortality expected for males in the general public. The excess mortality for men aged 25 to 34 was an astonishing 1,200 percent. For those 35 to 54, the excess mortality declined to 550 percent, and for men 55 to 64 years of age, the mortality was only twice that of the normal-weight

men in the general population. Excess mortality associated with obesity is greatly increased in younger persons and, not surprisingly, excess mortality is substantially higher in grossly obese persons.

Recent studies have shown that the weight range associated with lowest mortality increases with age in both men and women (National Institutes of Health Consensus Conference, 1985), indicating that excess weight later in life is not as harmful as excess weight earlier in life. In fact, Mattila and colleagues (1986) report that survival among people 65 years of age or older is greater in individuals with a higher body mass index.

The effects of too many pounds may be more important in younger persons than in those who pick up extra weight later in life. In several studies, men who became overweight early in life had more cardiovascular problems later. For example, Abraham and his colleagues (1971) related the changes in weight status between childhood and adult life to the incidence of hypertension, cardiovascular, and renal disease in 715 males. Childhood weight was determined from school weights recorded when these men were 9 to 13 years old. They were then reweighed at an average age of 48. The highest incidence of hypertension and cardiovascular-renal disease was recorded in men with the lowest childhood weight who had become overweight as adults.

In a similar study, Dr. Avia Must (1992) of the Human Nutrition Research Center on Aging at Tufts University in Boston related weight status in adolescence to morbidity and mortality later in life. Men and women who initially participated in the Harvard Growth Study of 1922–1935 were studied. For subjects who had died, cause of death was determined from death certificates. The average age of subjects at follow-up was 73 years. About 52 percent of living subjects who were overweight as adolescents were still overweight at follow-up.

Male subjects overweight in adolescence had twice the death rate as lean adolescents, regardless of adult weight. Death rate from coronary heart disease, atherosclerotic cerebrovascular disease, stroke, and colon cancer was higher in these subjects. In contrast, women overweight in adolescence did not have higher overall or disease-specific death rates compared with women who were lean as adolescents. However, overweight women had a 1.6 higher incidence of arthritis.

Insurance studies and data from the ongoing Framingham study have shown that losing excess pounds may prolong life. In both men and women who successfully lose and maintain a lower weight during their lifetimes, mortality rates were reduced to within normal limits for sex and age. In the Framingham study, reducing body weight by 10 percent decreased incidence of coronary artery disease by 20 percent (Kannel, 1986).

PROSPECTIVE STUDIES

The Framingham Study

The Framingham study is perhaps one of the longest and best publicized surveys of the effects of nutrition and weight on health, particularly cardiovascular health. For over 26 years, more than 5,000 residents of Framingham, Massachusetts, were examined, tested, and clinically followed in an effort to find epidemiologic clues to the development of cardiovascular disease and other illnesses (Hubert et al., 1983).

After following the population for 26 years, 870 men and 688 women in the Framingham study had died. Relative weight at the time a person entered the study was found to be an independent predictor of cardiovascular disease, particularly in women. Researchers were able to predict the incidence of coronary artery disease and the death rate from coronary artery disease. The likelihood of developing heart failure in men was predicted from the initial degree of overweight. The initial predictive power of being overweight was independent of such factors as age, cholesterol level, systolic blood pressure, cigarette smoking, or glucose intolerance.

The researchers concluded that obesity is an important long-term predictor of cardiovascular disease, particularly in younger persons. In women, only age and blood pressure level were more powerful predictors. Among the 2,223 men in the study, the lowest mortality over 30 years of age occurred at a relative weight of 100 percent to 109 percent of the Metropolitan Life weight table for 1959, for both smokers and nonsmokers (Metropolitan Life Insurance Company, 1982). The Framingham researchers estimated that if everyone were at their optimal weight, there would be 25 percent fewer cases of coronary disease, and 35 percent fewer cases of congestive heart failure and brain infarction.

The American Cancer Society Study

The American Cancer Society, published the results of a prospective study of more than 750,000 persons reviewed between 1959 and 1972 (Simonson, 1983). In this study, relative death rates among subgroups of people whose weights deviated above or below average established body weights were compared with the death rates for a group with an average weight 90 to 109 percent above average.

As weight increased, the overall mortality rate spiraled upward. Because of the special interest this organization has in smoking, the subjects were also divided into smokers and nonsmokers. A smoker of normal body weight has an increased mortality rate comparable to that of a nonsmoker with a body mass index (BMI) of 30 to 35 kg/m^2. The BMI is determined by taking the body weight (in kg), divided by the square of the height (in meters), or BMI=kg/m^2. As we'll see in the next chapter, the BMI is one of the better means of correlating body fat and body density. There is no increase in deaths until the BMI reaches 25 kg/m^2. These findings were similar to those of the build study (Build and Blood Pressure study, 1959) and the Framingham study. Excess weight also had a profound effect upon death from diabetes mellitus and gallbladder disease.

Cancer could also be correlated with weight status. As the BMI increased, there was an increase in cancer deaths, although the effect was much slighter than other causes of death. Overweight males had significantly higher rates of prostatic and colorectal cancer. For women, overweight could be correlated with a much higher incidence of cancer of the gallbladder, breasts, cervix, endometrium, uterus, and ovary.

The Gothenberg and Norwegian Studies

Two Scandinavian studies have also given us some interesting data about the effect of overweight on health. In some ways, the Gothenberg study (Lapidus et al., 1984) can be compared to the Framingham study. The Gothenberg study was a large prospective study conducted in Gothenberg, a city of about 450,000 people in southwest Sweden. This study has added some very important information about the health consequences of moderate obesity.

In men, the BMI and ratio of waist-to-hip circumference were positively correlated in those who eventually developed strokes. Men in the highest tertile (3 percent) for waist/hip ratio and the highest tertile for BMI had a 20.8 percent risk for developing strokes compared to a 5.6 percent risk for men in the lowest tertile of the BMI and the waist-to-hips ratio.

The greatest risk of cardiovascular disease was reported in men who had the highest waist-to-hips ratio and the lowest BMI. In this case, having the proverbial "beer belly" and "love handles," or extra fat around the waist, was particularly risky for persons who weren't otherwise very overweight.

Among the 14,462 women from 38 to 60 years of age studied in Gothenberg, the 12-year age-specific

death rates for myocardial infarction, stroke, and death from all causes were related to the waist-to-hips fat ratio. At the highest quintile (5 percent), the relative risk of myocardial infarction was increased 8.2 times above that for persons in the lowest quintile.

For stroke and overall death rate, the relative risk increased 3.9 and 2.0 percent for those in the highest quintile for waist-to-hips circumference. When women in the top 5 percent of the waist-to-hips ratio were compared with the women in the lowest 5 percent of waist-to-hips ratio, it was found that the risk of myocardial infarction was increased 14.8 percent; the risk of having a stroke was increased 11.0 times, and the risk of dying was increased by 4.8 times. Increasing BMI and higher waist-to-hips ratio enhanced the risk of developing coronary artery disease.

The Norwegian study (Waaler, 1983) used a quite different technique to study a majority of the Norwegian population between 1963 and 1975. A nationwide x-ray screening program provided height and weight measurements for a large proportion of the people in Norway. A total of 1,717,000 men and women aged 15 to 90 were followed during the 12-year study. (By comparison, the 1987 population of Norway was 4,165,000.)

Minimal mortality rates for men and women occurred at a BMI of 23. There was a steep increase in death rate when the BMI was lower than 23. Between 23 and 27 BMI the relative mortality was stable. As the BMI increased above 27, there was a curvilinear increase in excess mortality.

There was also a strong negative association between mortality and height; greater height was associated with lower mortality. Shorter persons were more likely to die from tuberculosis, obstructive lung disease, and cancer of the stomach and lung.

Among overweight people, the principal causes of death were cerebrovascular disease, cardiovascular diseases, diabetes mellitus, and cancer of the colon. It was concluded that excess mortality could have been reduced by 15 percent if all subjects had been closer to their ideal weights.

The Nurses' Health Study

Data of risk factors for coronary heart disease in women are sparse. The Nurses' Health Study (Manson, 1990) examined the influence of current obesity, relative weight at the age of 18, and intervening weight gain on subsequent risk for fatal and nonfatal coronary heart disease. This large-scale prospective study included 115,886 healthy females who were also registered nurses. Follow-up was over an eight-year period.

Subjects were divided into five weight categories based on body mass index. After eight years, obesity was shown to be a strong risk factor for fatal and non-fatal coronary heart disease (Figure 3.1). Subjects in the highest weight category had 3.3 times the risk for heart disease as subjects in the lowest weight category. In the heaviest women, 70 percent of coronary heart disease events were attributable to obesity. Even mild to moderate overweight was associated with increased risk of coronary heart disease.

Current body weight was more predictive of coronary heart disease than weight at age 18. Furthermore, weight gain between age 18 and current age substantially increased coronary risk. Nurses who gained 10 to 19.9kg (22 to 44 pounds) during adulthood had a 60 percent greater risk of coronary heart disease than nurses who gained less than 3kg (6 pounds). Nurses who gained 20 to 34.9 kg (44 to 77 pounds) had over a 200 percent greater risk of coronary heart disease.

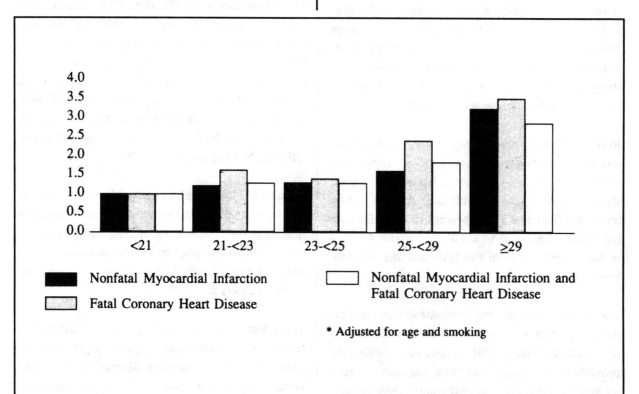

Figure 3.1 Relative risks of nonfatal myocardial infarction, fatal coronary heart disease, and nonfatal myocardial infarction and fatal coronary heart disease combined, according to body mass index.*

Source: Manson, J.E., Colditz, G. A., Stampfer, M.J., et al. A prospective study of obesity and risk of coronary heart disease in women. Reprinted by permission of *The New England Journal of Medicine*, 322, 882–889, 1990.

CARDIOVASCULAR DISEASE

Atherosclerosis develops early in life and progresses as we age. Fatty materials, or lipids, carried in the blood as cholesterol are deposited in the lining of arteries and form rough plaques that slowly increase in size. With time, the plaque builds up and gradually reduces the opening in the artery through which blood flows. The artery can become completely blocked, cutting off the blood supply to the area it serves. If this happens to be a portion of the brain, a stroke occurs. If it is a coronary artery, a heart attack may follow.

The heart receives its blood supply by coronary arteries. Three of the primary coronary arteries are the right coronary artery, the left anterior descending and the circumflex, each about the size of a pencil. If these arteries become clogged with atherosclerotic plaque, they will narrow and eventually close so that insufficient blood, carrying oxygen and nutrients, is supplied to the heart. The heart, of course, is a muscle as well as one of the most efficient mechanical devices in the body. It functions beautifully as long as its blood supply continues normally.

Atherosclerosis isn't just a disease of Americans or of the twentieth century. Signs of atherosclerosis have been found from modern-day autopsies on Egyptian mummies. Leonardo da Vinci attempted to relate pathological changes in the coronary arteries to clinical symptoms, such as angina pectoris, and described sclerotic blood vessels in the sixteenth century (Mayer et al., 1954).

Atherosclerosis tends to affect large and medium-sized arteries, usually the aorta and the iliac, femoral, coronary, and cerebral arteries. In terms of public health, myocardial infarction and stroke are the most common lethal diseases in the U.S. and most other developed nations. Cardiovascular disease is responsible for more than half of all deaths (Grundy, 1983).

A disease that starts early in life. Heart disease begins in the teenage years. By the time a man is 20 years old, the odds are that three of his coronary arteries are at least 20 percent closed. A typical healthy 30-year-old woman has 20 percent closure of one coronary artery. This 10-year lag behind men in development of heart disease continues for women until menopause, when the level of heart disease catches up. It may be shocking, but an average, healthy 35-year-old man will probably have 50 percent closure of all three coronary arteries. It's very difficult to detect such progression of disease except on autopsy, because the heart is such an efficient machine. Even if all three arteries are 65 percent closed, it is common for a man to pass even the most vigorous treadmill test without any signs of heart disease (Simonson, 1983).

The fact that the process of atherosclerosis begins in the teenage years wasn't generally known until the Korean War. Dr. William Enos (1953) was the first to report this astonishing fact, based on autopsies performed on 300 American soldiers killed during the war. In 77 percent of these men, there was gross evidence of coronary disease, ranging from slight thickening of the intima of the arteries to complete occlusion of one or more of the main coronary branches. The average age of these men was 22 years, and the average amount of arterial closure was 20 percent. However, in at least 10 young men, the arteries were 90 to 100 percent closed; thus, they probably would have died of heart attacks had they not been killed in combat.

Dr. Enos places the blame for the early development of atherosclerosis squarely on the American diet. He came to this theory after he performed autopsies on male Japanese soldiers 20 to 30 years old. In marked contrast to his findings in young American soldiers, he found no significant signs of atherosclerosis in the Japanese men. These men had eaten low-fat diets composed primarily of fish, rice, fruits and vegetables, rather than the high-fat diets the young Americans had grown up eating.

As Dr. Myron Winick (1985) notes, atherosclerosis is exclusively a disease of man. Man is the only member of the animal kingdom that develops heart disease. Under normal conditions, no animal develops anything evenly remotely like closure of the arteries. Even under laboratory settings devised to simulate human conditions, very few animals can be induced to develop atherosclerosis. In addition, atherosclerosis is almost never seen in primitive societies.

Atherosclerosis can also be blamed in some part on our genes, for the tendency to heart disease does run in families. For most Americans the role of genetic background in development of heart disease is not as important as the impact of our lifestyles.

Atherosclerosis not only produces the dramatic events of stroke or myocardial infarction, but also can affect smaller vessels, leading to senility, confusion, loss of memory, and incoherence.

Risk Factors

Several factors beyond our control influence the risk of developing atherosclerosis and subsequent cardiovascular diseases. Males have a higher risk of cardiovascular disease than females, and risk increases with age for both males and females. Black individuals have a higher risk than white individuals. Individuals with a strong family history of cardiovascular disease are also at greater risk of developing the disease.

In addition to the factors we cannot control, other factors that we can control influence the risk of atherosclerosis and cardiovascular disease. Five major, modifiable risk factors for atherosclerosis include high blood cholesterol levels (hyperlipidemia), high blood pressure (hypertension), cigarette smoking, diabetes, and obesity. Although the type A personality pattern characterized by aggressiveness, ambi-

tion, impatience, and a chronic sense of time urgency also used to be considered a risk factor; many recent studies have cast doubt on this theory. In fact, individuals tending toward a type A personality may recover from a heart attack better than more relaxed individuals tending toward a type B personality (Case, 1985).

Cigarette smoking. Increased risk of atherosclerosis, in the form of stroke, myocardial infarction, and intermittent claudication is seen in male smokers in contrast to nonsmokers. Women who smoke have an increased incidence of intermittent claudication as well.

By the time a male smoker reaches 45 years of age, his excess risk of atherosclerosis is about 70 percent. At autopsy, the degree of atherosclerosis can be very closely correlated with previous smoking. In addition to narrowing of the coronary arteries, smaller intramyocardial arteries have shown fibromuscular intimal thickening. These changes are not only related to the number of cigarettes smoked, but can also be found in persons who smoke cigars and pipes.

Sudden death is a clinical event frequently associated with cigarette smoking. Stopping smoking, even after years of heavy smoking, can sharply reduce this risk. Scientists have looked to the levels of carboxyhemoglobin for clues to sudden death. They have found that levels of carboxyhemoglobin are significantly increased in smokers. Men from 30 to 69 years of age who reach carboxyhemoglobin levels of about 15 percent on a regular basis have a twenty-fold greater incidence of atherosclerotic vascular disease and events such as myocardial infarction, angina pectoris, and intermittent claudication, compared to nonsmokers or smokers who have carboxyhemoglobin levels of 3 percent or lower (Aronow, 1980). The problem is that a narrowed coronary artery may not be able to deliver the 20 percent increase in blood flow needed to offset the decreased availability of oxygen from blood containing 5 percent carboxyhemoglobin.

As discussed earlier, results of the Framingham study (Hubert, 1983) and other studies show that obesity is an independent risk factor for cardiovascular disease. Obesity also increases risk for cardiovascular disease through its effects on other cardiovascular risk factors such as hyperlipidemia, hypertension, and type II diabetes. Upper body obesity in particular contributes to these risk factors (Manson, 1990).

Two ongoing studies are taking a look at the impact of reducing risk factors for atherosclerosis. The Multiple Risk Factor Intervention Trial (MRFIT) and Hypertension Detection and Follow-up Program (HDFP) were designed to reduce cholesterol, blood pressure, and cigarette smoking, to see if this could have an impact upon coronary heart disease.

The MRFIT study (Podell, 1983) was designed to see if not just one but several risk factors could be reduced and decrease the incidence of cardiovascular disease. Special efforts were made to intervene to reduce the risk of hypertension, smoking, and hyperlipidemia. The study involved 12,866 men aged 35 to 57 who were free of complications of atherosclerosis but who were at high risk for cardiovascular disease because of high cholesterol intake, high blood pressure, and smoking habits. The men were randomized into two groups. One group was given special intervention, including dietary advice, stepped-care for hypertension, and counseling on smoking cessation. The second group was given typical care in their own communities.

After seven years of follow-up, the men in both groups had significant decreases in serum cholesterol, diastolic blood pressure, and cigarette smoking. However, the decreases were much greater in the special-intervention group than in the men who received typical care.

Although the coronary heart disease and cardiovascular disease mortality were less in the special-intervention group than in the group that received typical care, the differences weren't statistically different. Certain subgroups of men did benefit more than others, with the exception of some men who had an unfavorable response to some of the antihypertensive drugs used in the program. The special intervention and regular-care groups both benefited greatly by stopping smoking, which led to significantly lower rates of coronary artery disease.

The HDFP study (1979) was designed to see if blood pressure could be lowered and, if so, whether deaths due to heart attacks and stroke could be decreased. The study involved 10,940 hypertensive men and women aged 30 to 69, who were randomly assigned either to routine care in the community for their high blood pressure or to special clinics, at which care was designed to bring their blood pressure back to specific goal levels. In this way, the design was very similar to that used for the MRFIT study.

After five years of follow-up, it was found that patients who received goal-focused clinical care had lower blood pressure levels than patients who were given routine care. In addition, there was a 17 percent reduction in the overall death rate, a 45 percent reduction in the stroke death rate, and a 26 percent reduction in the heart attack death rate, compared to the rates in those receiving usual care. These changes were also present in patients who had been considered "mild hypertensives."

This study conclusively showed that patients with mild hypertension could benefit from therapy. The heart attack death rate among people with less severe hypertension was 46 percent lower in the goal-focused clinical care patients than in those receiving regular medical care.

HYPERLIPIDEMIA

Risk for heart disease increases with increasing serum cholesterol levels in a curvilinear fashion, with risk sharply rising at cholesterol levels above 240mg/dl. Cholesterol contributes to atherosclerosis and cardiovascular disease by clogging blood vessels and blocking blood flow.

Cholesterol is manufactured in the body and is also present in food. Serum levels are determined by the availability of cholesterol from these two sources. Most of the endogenous cholesterol is manufactured by the liver, then transported to other organs as needed. Many of the hormones produced by the adrenal gland are made from cholesterol. The insulation around nerve sheaths in the brain is mostly cholesterol. The gallbladder uses cholesterol to produce bile. Cholesterol is such an important ingredient, according to Dr. Winick (1985), that it is reabsorbed from the bile when it is secreted into the intestines. Cholesterol is essential for life and becomes a health hazard only when it occurs in excess amounts. The body regulates the amount of cholesterol, producing less if more is provided by the diet. This protective mechanism can be overwhelmed when people consume very large amounts of cholesterol or saturated fats.

Saturated fats are those fats found in meat and dairy products. Polyunsaturated fats, found in vegetable sources, are believed to lower blood cholesterol levels.

Cholesterol is transported in the blood attached to proteins, forming lipoproteins. Most cholesterol is carried by low-density lipoproteins, or LDLs. LDL has been of the greatest interest to researchers, for several reasons. Levels of total serum cholesterol almost always correlate with high levels of LDL cholesterol. A small amount of cholesterol is carried by another protein, which has a much higher density and is termed high-density lipoprotein, or HDL. A higher amount of HDL is more desirable because it is thought that this type of cholesterol actually comes from arterial plaques and reduces the amount of atherosclerosis.

LDL is only one of a large group of plasma proteins, the lipoproteins, that are important in transportation of cholesterol. Cholesterol accumulates in smooth muscle and other cells in atherosclerotic lesions or plaques. New studies have shown that abnormalities in the cell's receptors for LDLs produce elevated blood lipids and contribute to development of atherosclerosis. Hyperlipidemia is not always easy to define. It is often said that the normal blood-cholesterol level is about 250mg per ml. It may be far better to aim for a level below this, one closer to 200mg per ml.

High blood cholesterol is more prevalent among overweight individuals than among lean individuals. Thirty-two percent of overweight men have high blood cholesterol levels as compared to 22 percent of lean men (National Heart, Lung, and Blood Institute, 1993). The figures are similar for women. Thirty-eight percent of overweight women compared with 25 percent of lean women have high blood cholesterol levels. Data from the Framingham study and the Second National Health and Nutrition Examination Survey confirm that mean serum cholesterol levels increase with increasing body weight.

HYPERTENSION

The prevalence of high blood pressure in overweight individuals is more than twice that of lean individuals (National Heart, Lung, and Blood Institute, 1993). Fifty-five percent of obese men have high blood pressure compared with 27 percent of lean men. Fifty-two percent of obese women have high blood pressure compared with 19 percent of lean women. Similar to high blood cholesterol levels, the mean level of both systolic and diastolic blood pressure increases in linear fashion with increasing body weight (National Institutes of Health, 1993).

High blood pressure accelerates atherosclerosis. A person with a systolic blood pressure greater than 160 mmHg or a diastolic greater than 95 mmHg has a fivefold increased risk of coronary heart disease, compared to persons with normal blood pressure. Hypertension poses the greatest risk factor for clinical disease in persons older than 45 years of age, and is a strong predictor of brain infarction.

The relationship of hypertension to obesity has been recognized for many years. More than 37 million American adults are believed to have high blood pressure (American Heart Association, 1987). For those who know they are hypertensive, many are untreated and many others have blood pressure that is inadequately controlled. Hypertension is well nicknamed "the silent killer," because it often produces no outward signs and if not controlled can kill with little warning. The reason for elevated blood pressure isn't known in as many as 90 percent of those affected. However, it is easily detected and usually can be controlled with diet and medication.

As blood circulates throughout the body, it produces a certain pressure within the arteries and veins. The heart initially causes the pressure as it forces blood out through its ventricles to the aorta, then through the arterial system. Blood pressure is never static, but oscillates between high and low volume, depending on whether the heart is contracting or relaxing. During contraction, blood is forced out under maximum pressure, or systolic pressure. During relaxation, and while the ventricles refill with blood, the arterial pressure falls to a lower level, or diastolic pressure. Contractions last a relatively short time, so that the arterial system is exposed to diastolic pressure most of the time.

The two values, systolic and diastolic pressure, are usually recorded in the normal range of about 120/80 mmHg. High blood pressure is defined as a systolic pressure of 140 mmHg or higher or diastolic pressure 90 mmHg or above. High diastolic pressure is thought to be more dangerous because the arteries are exposed to this level of pressure for a greater length of time.

Hypertension promotes deposition of cholesterol from the blood into the arterial walls and thus it is a primary risk factor for developing atherosclerosis. High blood pressure can also cause aneurysms and rupture of blood vessels. When small vessels leading to the brain develop an aneurysm or rupture, cerebral hemorrhage (a stroke) can occur. This same prolonged high pressure can rupture small vessels in the kidneys, ultimately leading to kidney failure, and add stress on the heart, leading to heart failure.

Hypertension is much more common in blacks than whites. It runs in families in both groups. Blood pressure also rises with age in the U.S. For many years, this gradual increase in pressure with age was thought to be normal. In other cultures, such as Polynesians, or Eskimos in Greenland, blood pressure doesn't change with age. In fact, hypertension is almost nonexistent in these cultures. In the U.S., it is estimated that as many as 30 percent of people have hypertension. This percentage is even higher in China and Japan (Frohlich, 1983).

The one similarity between diets in the U.S., China, and Japan, is that the diets all contain high amounts of sodium. A number of studies have tracked the increase in blood pressure in people who move from a setting with little or no salt in their diet to those with a high salt content. For example, the Samburu, a tribal group from northern Kenya, ordinarily exist on a diet of meat and milk, with very little sodium. When a group of the young tribesmen were drafted into the Kenyan army, their dietary intake of sodium increased by five times (Frolich, 1983). During the second year of service in the army, their blood pressures began to inch upward and continued to increase for the six years they served in the army.

Some of the best information about the role of diet on hypertension comes from studies of laboratory animals. Just as in humans, only certain strains of rats will develop hypertension, no matter how much salt they are given. Even in susceptible animals, however, hypertension occurs only when dietary salt levels are increased.

Once hypertension develops in a laboratory animal it will not automatically go back to normal levels, even though the high-sodium diet is changed and the animal returned to its original diet. As Dr. Winick (1985) explains, sodium is an element essential for life and is present in all cells and all body fluids. The body must regulate the amount of sodium it contains, primarily through the kidneys. When too much sodium is available, the kidney does not reabsorb the excess, which increases the amount excreted by the kidneys. When too little sodium is available, the kidney filters it from the blood, and reabsorbs it. In the kidney, the blood is filtered through the glomerulus, a collection of small arteries. The higher the pressure on these arteries, to a certain level, the more efficient the filtration. (Note - Too high pressure can destroy the glomerulus). The kidney then secretes a number of hormones that assist the brain in raising and lowering blood pressure.

Once the arteries have been contracted for a long time, they become more fixed and will not relax as easily when salt intake increases. Thus, genetic make-up, which determines how well the kidney regulates sodium intake through hormonal response, determines whether people are prone to develop hypertension. In some people, slight increases in sodium in the diet will evoke this response. These individuals are susceptible to high blood pressure. In other people, even large increases in sodium intake can be handled easily by the kidney without increasing blood pressure. As the kidney ages, it

becomes less efficient as a sodium filter, and thus it raises blood pressure in response to lower and lower salt intakes. Because so much of the daily diet is high in sodium, it isn't unusual for hypertension to develop with age. In contrast, in other societies where dietary intake of sodium is much less, this pattern is never seen.

Overconsumption of calories is a second factor that is related to hypertension. The heavier a person is, the greater his or her chances are of developing hypertension. This risk is independent of sodium consumption. At any given sodium intake level, an obese person is more prone to develop hypertension than a thinner person.

When weight is lost, blood pressure usually drops. For example, hypertension nearly vanished among people who had great caloric deprivation during World War II. Dr. Bray (1985) notes that 50 to 80 percent of persons who lose weight also have a reduction in blood pressure. One might immediately think this is merely a reflection of lower sodium levels in the diet, but studies have shown that blood pressure fell even when the sodium content of the diet was kept constant. Tuck (1981) and his colleagues have suggested that lower caloric intake may reduce blood pressure by lowering the activity of the sympathetic nervous system.

Other dietary factors that may influence blood pressure include potassium, calcium, magnesium, and dietary fat intake (National Institutes of Health, 1993). High potassium intake may protect against developing high blood pressure. Calcium deficiency may make a person more at risk of developing high blood pressure. Preliminary studies suggest that low dietary magnesium intake may also increase risk for high blood pressure, though these studies need to be confirmed. A certain type of fat, the omega-3 fatty acids found in rich concentrations in fatty fish such as salmon, mackerel, and haddock, may also help lower blood pressure.

DIABETES

Diabetes, one of the most serious yet relatively common problems in modern times, results from a deficiency of insulin—a hormone produced by the pancreas. There are two main forms of diabetes. Type I diabetes, also called insulin-dependent diabetes mellitus (IDDM), usually occurs in childhood and is characterized by a complete inability to manufacture insulin in the body. Type II diabetes, also called non-insulin-dependent diabetes (NIDDM), usually develops later in life and is characterized by varying ability to make insulin and resistance to the action of insulin in the body.

Type I diabetes is due to an absolute lack of insulin. The mechanisms within the pancreas that produce insulin are damaged and can no longer produce insulin. This severe type of diabetes must be treated quickly with insulin, which the patient must take for the rest of his life. The disease is definitely caused by a genetic component. The cells within the pancreas that produce insulin are selectively destroyed by what appears to be a viral infection. Unless the young patient is detected and treated quickly, he will rapidly become ill and die. There are no dietary changes that can stop this type of diabetes, but the child must constantly watch his diet.

Type II diabetes also results from a deficiency of insulin. In this form of diabetes, however, the pancreas may produce enough insulin, but the body requires even larger supplies. The pancreas simply can't keep up with the demand. Type II diabetes usually develops after the age of 50 and tends to run in families. Some groups, such as Ashkenazie Jews, African Americans, and American Indians are at greater risk of developing diabetes. Dietary modification can have a powerful impact upon this type of diabetes.

Insulin is produced by special cells, called beta cells, which are found in small clumps between the ducts of the pancreas, called the islets of Langerhans. The insulin produced by the beta cells is secreted directly into the bloodstream and is then carried to all tissues in the body. The beta cells have molecular arm-like protrusions from their surface into which insulin molecules fit and are bound to the cell surface. These receptors are specific for insulin. Usually there are more receptor sites than insulin molecules. As the demand for insulin increases, more insulin is produced, and insulin molecules immediately become fixed to a receptor and are quickly absorbed by a cell. If any of the receptors aren't working properly, the pancreas is called upon to produce more insulin.

Once the insulin enters the cell, it helps glucose, the body's main energy source, move from the blood into the tissues. Here the glucose will be stored as fuel, as fat, or as the complex carbohydrate glycogen. In the case of fat cells, insulin allows glucose to enter and be converted to fat. When we eat too many calories, our body stores them as fat. To do this, more insulin is needed than when caloric intake is lower. To build up or to maintain fat stores, an obese person needs more insulin than a lean person needs.

If the beta cells can supply the body's need for insulin, the body will function normally. If they cannot do so, an individual develops an insulin deficiency and the symptoms of diabetes will appear. In some people, the beta cells can easily make the added insulin. In others, the cells just can't keep up with the need.

In some persons at risk for diabetes, the disease doesn't develop until they are fairly elderly, 70 years of age or older. However, if enough strain is placed on the beta cells, such as with obesity, the disease may develop even sooner. People who have a genetic tendency to develop diabetes will do so at a much younger age if they are obese.

Diabetes is the third most frequent cause of death in the United States (Perri, 1992). Obesity is a strong risk factor for type II diabetes. About 80 percent of diabetics have type II diabetes. Of these individuals, 60 to 90 percent are obese. In fact, obesity is probably the single most important factor in the development of type II diabetes, and weight loss is the most important treatment goal.

About 60 percent of individuals with severe obesity eventually develop type II diabetes (Grundy, 1990). The longer the duration of obesity, the greater the risk of developing type II diabetes (Everhart, 1992).

Controlling obesity through diet can thus have a powerful effect upon diabetes. In one group studied by Drenick (1980), a number of obese men, none of whom had signs of diabetes, were followed for six years. During the six years of follow-up, frank diabetes began appearing in members of the group, until more than 40 percent had been affected by the disease. An additional 40 percent of these men had impaired glucose tolerance, meaning that during the six years of the study, more than 80 percent of the group had deterioration of glucose tolerance.

In another study, Toeller and colleagues (1982) reported following up 60 persons, including 11 men and 49 women. All the subjects were given glucose tolerance tests at the beginning of the study and again at two five-year intervals for 10 years. At the beginning of the study, five subjects were diabetic and remained diabetic during the study. The remaining 55 patients fell into groups with either normal or impaired glucose tolerance. At the end of 10 years, nine persons with initially normal glucose tolerance had become diabetic and seven had impaired glucose tolerance. Of the 29 persons who initially had impaired glucose tolerance, 14 had normal glucose tolerance five years later, and four kept their status for at least 10 years. All those subjects who had normal glucose tolerance also had a steady decrease in the amount of overweight during the 10-year period, falling from an initial value of 68 percent

overweight, to 62 percent overweight at five years, and 53 percent overweight at 10 years.

At all ages, diabetes is associated with atherosclerosis. In premenopausal women, coronary insufficiency is 20 times more common in diabetic women than in nondiabetic women. When a myocardial infarction occurs in a man younger than 40, it is almost always found in a person who either has diabetes or a familial lipid disorder. Fifty percent of all diabetics die prematurely of myocardial infarctions.

Diabetes is also associated with high blood pressure. The resistance to insulin that commonly occurs in type II diabetes may explain the link between diabetes and high blood pressure. Insulin resistance may also explain the link between diabetes and hyperlipidemia and cardiovascular disease (DeFronzo, 1991). The mechanisms by which insulin resistance could trigger high blood pressure are not clearly understood, but could involve sodium retention in the body, overactivity of the sympathetic nervous system, disturbances in ion transport across membranes, or proliferation of vascular smooth-muscle cells.

High insulin levels in the body and insulin resistance promote hyperlipidemia by causing the body to manufacture more very low-density lipoproteins, leading to higher levels of triglycerides and low-density lipoproteins in the blood. High levels of insulin are also known to promote atherosclerosis independent of insulin's effects on blood fat levels.

It is easy to see, from the few studies we've mentioned, that obesity and overweight can have a powerful effect on the development and course of diabetes. Weight loss has a powerful impact on improving glucose tolerance and insulin secretion. Drenick (1980) studied three groups of subjects before and after they lost weight, and again after they regained some of their weight. When glucose tolerance was initially normal, the insulin response to glucose improved.

CANCER

The risk of cancer increases with increasing body weight. In a large-scale study of 750,000 subjects conducted by the American Cancer Society (Lew, 1979), risk of cancer was increased in both obese men and women, particularly in those over 40 percent of ideal weight, compared with their lean counterparts. In obese men, cancer of the colon, rectum, prostate, pancreas, and stomach was increased. In obese women, cancer of the endometrium, breast, gallbladder, cervix, and ovary was increased.

The death rate from cancer for men 40 percent or more overweight was one-third higher than for men of average weight. The death rate for cancer among women 40 percent or more overweight was 55 percent higher than for women of average weight.

Obesity increases risk of endometrial cancer during the premenopausal as well as post menopausal years. Women who weigh more than 30 percent of ideal weight have twice the risk of endometiral cancer, whereas women who weigh more than 40 percent of ideal weight have four times the risk. In contrast, the risk for breast cancer increases with obesity only after menopause.

Obese people have increased levels of prolactin, androgens, estrogens, and cortisol. Several studies have singled out estrogen as having a role in development of cancers of the reproductive system, such as endometrial, cervical, breast and ovarian cancer. Adipose tissue is the major site of estrogen formation.

Breast cancer is the most common cancer that strikes American women and is a leading cause of death in the U.S. In fact, American women experi-

ence a far greater incidence of breast cancer than women in other countries. Scientists who have tried to find a common link to this type of cancer have come up with only one possibility: a diet high in fat. They have found that the more fat a population consumes, no matter how highly developed or primitive the country is, the higher the incidence of breast cancer.

As we mentioned, obese persons have increased levels of certain hormones. Because breast cancer is common in women and uncommon in men, studies suggest that a hormonal imbalance in some as yet unknown way promotes breast cancer.

Colon cancer is very common is the U.S., and its incidence is increasing. A recent study suggests that overweight during middle age or young adulthood increases risk of developing colon cancer (Lee, 1992). The best correlation of cancer of the colon is with a diet high in fat. Unlike breast cancer, men are just as likely to have colon cancer as women. Theories about development of colon cancer suggest that a high-fat diet changes the normal bacterial flora of the large intestine. Bacteria easily survive and easily transform the fat into other products, some of which may act as carcinogens.

Low fiber in the diet may also be an important factor. Much can be read and heard about fiber, which is the portion of the carbohydrate within food that is indigestible and not absorbed by the body. Fiber can be derived from plants, such as the bran of certain grains, and from the skin and fleshy portion of some fruits and vegetables. Dietary fiber also attracts water to it. As fiber passes through the gastrointestinal tract, it will soften the stool, making it easier to pass. The softer the stool, the faster it can be propelled through the large intestine and the less time it comes in contact with the wall of the intestine.

The value of fiber was first noted when scientists reported that certain African tribes who ate large amounts of fiber had virtually no cases of colon cancer. The theory (Connor, 1986) is that the rapid movement of fiber through the gastrointestinal tract keeps the fiber and any cancer-inducing chemicals in it from coming into contact with the intestinal wall.

Obese women have a slightly higher incidence of uterine cancer than lean women; this is particularly true for women who have been obese since childhood. One study (Lew, 1979), for example, reported that uterine cancer was 1.5 times more common in women who have been obese since adolescence than in those who are not obese.

In general, some people are at greater risk of developing cancer than others, due to family history, sex, and race. Here are a few examples:

The risk of developing breast cancer is greater for persons with the following factors:

- Caucasian
- Family history
- Female
- Women of higher socioeconomic status (due to high fat in the diet?)
- Later onset of menopause
- Nulliparas
- Primiparas over 35 years of age
- Early onset of menarche

The risk of developing uterine cancer is greater in women with the following characteristics:

- Obesity, especially during adolescence
- Late onset of menopause
- Exogenous estrogens

Much more study needs to be done to try to understand the dietary elements that may be at work in producing cancer. For the time being, however, it is clear that obesity and a high-fat diet do contribute to the development of certain types of cancer.

PULMONARY PROBLEMS

Obese persons have a number of problems with pulmonary function, ranging from general respiratory disorders to the extreme case of the Pickwickian syndrome. The work of breathing is increased when considerable additional weight is carried on the chest wall. In addition, excessive fatty tissue also increases the complexity of getting oxygen to all the tissues of the body. As a result of reduced oxygenation, obese persons have lower tolerance levels for exercise and may even have difficulty in normal breathing, particularly with a respiratory infection.

The Pickwickian syndrome, which was named after Dickens' character Joe, a fat boy in *The Pickwick Papers,* is marked by hypoventilation, somnolence, and obesity. Losing weight is essential for treatment of the Pickwickian syndrome, as well as a patient's suffering from congestive heart failure.

Individuals who have significant changes in pulmonary function are often significantly obese and have other respiratory or cardiovascular problems. When Dr. Bray (1976) and his colleagues studied 29 obese women and 14 obese men, they found there was a progressive decrease in expiratory reserve volume as the weight-to-height ratio increased. Vital capacity, residual volume, and diffusion capacity remained fairly constant until the patients became massively obese, or until their weight-height ratio exceeded 1.0.

Obese people may also have problems with respiratory muscle function and disturbed ventilation and perfusion. This is seen most often in the Pickwickian syndrome, often called the obesity-hypoventilation syndrome. Ongoing studies are attempting to show that this problem is largely due to sleep apnea. For example, Sharp (1983) and co-workers believe that the hypoxemia and hypercapnia that occur during part of the day may eventually adversely affect control of ventilation during the rest of the day. Hypoxia that occurs with obstructive or mixed sleep apnea produces hypoxia that worsens as obesity advances. A dangerous cycle is set in motion; hypoxia blunts the hyperoxic drive, sleep is disturbed, and compensatory sleep occurs during the day. In time, hypoxemia is followed by hypercapnia, which may eventually lead to cor pulmonale and right-sided heart failure.

GALLBLADDER DISEASE

At least 500,000 persons undergo treatment for gallstones each year (National Institutes of Health, 1987). Gallbladder disease and digestive disease in general are more common in obese persons (Kato 1992). Digestive diseases are 40 percent above the normal level in persons who are 15 to 35 percent overweight and nearly 150 percent above normal in those who are 65 percent or more overweight. The American Cancer Society study also showed that overweight persons are more likely than normal-weight persons to die from digestive disease.

The phrase so often used to describe persons at risk of developing gallstones, "Fair, Fat, Female, and Forty," is fairly accurate. Overweight women aren't alone in their increased risk of developing gallstones. Sturdevant (1973) found that the body weight of men without gallstones was significantly less than in men with gallstones.

In any age group, the frequency of gallbladder disease increases with the level of body weight. For women 25 to 34 years of age who are 100 percent or

more overweight, 18 percent had gallbladder disease, compared to nearly 35 percent of the women aged 45 to 55 who were 100 percent or more overweight. In this study (Friedman, 1966), 88 percent of the variation in frequency of gallbladder disease was accounted for by weight, age, and parity. Weight was by far the most important variable. Among younger women, or those 20 to 30 years old, those who were obese had six times the risk of developing gallbladder disease than women of normal weight. By age 60, nearly one-third of women will have developed gallbladder disease. Even the Framingham study showed that persons who were at least 20 percent above the median weight for their height had about twice the risk of developing gallbladder disease than those who were less than 90 percent of the median weight for height.

How does weight correlate with gallbladder disease? One explanation might be that such persons have increased cholesterol production and secretion. Dr. Bray (1985) points out that there are several reasons this may be the key. First, there is a significant correlation between the degree of fatness and cholesterol levels. Second, the cholesterol production rate is correlated with body weight; for every extra kilogram of body weight, cholesterol production is increased by 20 to 22mg per day. Third, when the bile from obese persons is examined, it is found that it is far more saturated with cholesterol than that in nonobese persons. Finally, he adds that hepatic secretion of cholesterol is higher before weight is lost than afterward. Thus, the increased biliary excretion of cholesterol among obese persons is probably the cause of the increased risk of gallstones.

OTHER PROBLEMS

Hirsutism and menstrual irregularities are much more common among obese women and can often be improved by weight loss. Overweight can also cause problems during pregnancy. Complications of toxemia and delivery can be reduced if weight is controlled, preferably before pregnancy occurs. Obese men may be troubled with infertility.

Persons with bone and joint disease are helped by weight reduction. Reducing weight takes the excess pressure off the skeletal system and helps improve mobility of the joints.

Obesity may be an important risk factor in the development of diverticular disease (Schauer, 1992). Obesity, excessive weight gain in young adulthood, and high blood pressure are also risk factors for the development of gout (Roubenoff, 1991).

METABOLIC IMPLICATIONS OF BODY FAT DISTRIBUTION

The type of obesity also influences health risks. Upper body obesity (excess fat more in the trunk and abdominal areas) is more dangerous than lower body obesity (excess fat more in the buttock and hip areas). A waist to hip ratio of above 0.85 for women and 0.95 for men is associated with hypertension, hyperlipidemia, diabetes, and increased coronary heart disease mortality (Despres, 1990). Women with central obesity are also at greater risk of breast cancer than women with lower body obesity (Schapira, 1990).

Fat deposits around major body organs may pose a greater strain on the body than fat in extremities. Also, fat deposits in the trunk and abdominal areas are more metabolically active than fat deposits in the lower body, promoting insulin resistance and its associated problems of high blood pressure, diabetes, abnormal blood lipid levels, and cardiovascular disease (Bjorntorp, 1991).

The next chapter defines obesity more closely according to current accepted standards. Clinical, anthropometric, and dietary assessment of the obese patient will be discussed from a nursing perspective.

EXAM QUESTIONS

Chapter 3

Questions 19-29

19. Compared with ideal body weight for height published in life insurance tables, individuals with the lowest mortality rates have body weight:

    a. slightly under ideal weight
    b. within 1% of ideal weight
    c. slightly above ideal weight
    d. 20% above ideal weight

20. How early does discrimination against heavy persons begin?

    a. in childhood
    b. in early adolescence
    c. in late adolescence
    d. in adulthood

21. Data from the Framingham study indicate:

    a. obesity is an independent risk factor for cardiovascular disease in men and women
    b. obesity is an independent risk factor for cardiovascular disease only in men
    c. obesity is an independent risk factor for cardiovascular disease only in women
    d. obesity is not an independent risk factor for cardiovascular disease

22. Which of the following is not a risk factor for atherosclerosis?

    a. male gender
    b. female gender
    c. cigarette smoking
    d. obesity

23. The prevalence of elevated blood cholesterol levels in obese as compared to non-obese individuals is:

    a. slightly lower
    b. about the same
    c. slightly higher in men only
    d. slightly higher in men and women

24. Obesity increases the risk of what type of cancer?

    a. skin cancer
    b. colon cancer
    c. thyroid cancer
    d. liver cancer

25. How early in life does atherosclerosis begin?

    a. after age 40
    b. after age 35
    c. in the 20's and 30's
    d. in adolescence

26. In the Nurses Health Study, subjects in the highest weight category had what risk of coronary heart disease compared with subjects in the lowest weight category?

    a. less risk
    b. the same risk
    c. three times the risk
    d. five times the risk

27. Compared with normal-weight individuals, the prevalence of high blood pressure in obese individuals is:

    a. twice as high
    b. twice as low
    c. the same
    d. five times as high

28. What type of obesity is most associated with metabolic impairments such as high blood pressure, type II diabetes, and high blood lipid levels?

    a. upper body obesity in males only
    b. upper body obesity in males and females
    c. lower body obesity in females only
    d. lower body obesity in males and females

29. About what percentage of individuals with type II diabetes are obese?

    a. 20%
    b. 40%
    c. 60%
    d. 50%

CHAPTER 4

ASSESSMENT OF THE OBESE PATIENT

CHAPTER OBJECTIVE

After studying this chapter, you will be able to describe the key elements of a comprehensive assessment of the obese patient.

LEARNING OBJECTIVES

After studying this chapter, you will be able to:

1. Take a baseline health history and identify parts of the medical assessment specific to obesity.

2. Define obesity using standard height for weight tables and body mass index measurements.

3. Specify alternative dietary assessment measures and indicate their uses.

4. Identify features of anorexia nervosa and bulimia.

INTRODUCTION

The first three chapters delineate the many different physical and environmental factors that contribute to obesity. The physical and psychological consequences of obesity also have been discussed. To devise effective intervention strategies, nurses and other health professionals must carefully assess diet, exercise, and medical and family history. This chapter describes the medical, anthropometric, psychosocial, and dietary assessment of obesity.

MEDICAL ASSESSMENT

Health History

In the initial interview, the nurse will want to obtain basic information about the patient, including a family health history and the patient's own health history.

Most clinics use their own history-taking form. A sample history form is presented here that includes most data required. This form acts as a baseline management summary for obese patients. It also singles out obesity-related health risks such as cardiovascular disease.

BASELINE MANAGEMENT SUMMARY

Patient's name _____

Date _____

Marital status

Single ___ Married ___ Divorced ___ Widowed ___

Patient's Characteristics and Health Habits

Age ____ Sex ____ Height ____

Weight ___ % of ideal weight ____

Impairments that would affect dietary change or counseling _____

Adapted from: National Institutes of Health (1987). *Heart to Heart, A Manual on Nutrition. Counseling for the Reduction of Cardiovascular Disease Risk Factors.* Bethesda, MD. p. 26.

FAMILY MEDICAL HISTORY

Is the patient's father living?

Yes ___ No ___ Unsure ___

If not, at what age did he die? ____

Cause _____

Is the patient's mother living?

Yes ___ No ___ Unsure ___

If not, at what age did she die? ____

Cause _____

How many brothers and sisters does patient have? _____

How many are living? ____

Do or did any of the brothers or sisters, mother or father, have any of the following medical problems? (Use M for mother, F for father, S for sister, B for brother.)

Hypertension _____

Diabetes _____

Overweight _____

Stroke _____

Hyperlipidemia _____

Type _____

Diet prescription _____

Does the spouse have a weight problem?

Yes ___ No ___

Describe the problem:

_____

Hypertension Yes ___ No ___

Diabetes Yes ___ No ___

Premature heart attack Yes ___ No ___

Stroke Yes ___ No ___

Hyperlipidemia Yes ___ No ___

Type _____

Diet prescription _____

PATIENT'S MEDICAL HISTORY

Lowest adult weight _____
Highest adult weight _____

Does the patient have any evidence of cardiovascular disease?

Yes _____   No _____

Date _____

Describe _____
_____

Hyperlipoproteinemia?

Yes ___   No ____

Type _____

Lipid-lowering medications _____

Hypertension? Yes ___   No ___

Medications _____

Potassium supplement _____

Uric acid medications _____

Diabetes? Yes ___   No ___

Medications _____

Hypothyroidism? Yes ___   No ___

Medications _____

Kidney disease? Yes ___   No ___
Liver disease? Yes ___   No ___

Medications _____

Alcohol abuse? Yes ___   No ___

Taking corticosteroids? Yes ___   No ___

Taking oral contraceptives? Yes ___   No ___

ECG changes or positive stress test? Yes ___ No ___

Taking nonprescription drugs? Yes ___   No ___

Kind _____

Baseline Blood Values   **Date**

Total cholesterol   _____   _____

LDL cholesterol   _____   _____

VLDL cholesterol   _____   _____

HDL cholesterol   _____   _____

Triglycerides   _____   _____

Glucose   _____   _____

Uric acid   _____   _____

Potassium   _____   _____

Other:_____

Baseline blood pressure: ___/___ _____

Other Characteristics

Does patient live with:

Family ___ Friends ___ Alone ___

Patient's occupation:

_____

Hours per week ____ Shift work? _____

Occupations of others in household:

_____

_____

_____

_____

Household income level:

Low ___ Middle ___ High ___

Receiving assistance? _____

Patient's education:

Finished high school? Yes ___ No ___

Finished college? Yes ___ No ___

Does patient speak English? Yes ___ No ___
Other _____

Does patient read English? Yes ___ No ___

Other _____

Does patient have a seeing, hearing, or other impairment? Yes ___ No ___

Specify _____

If yes, does patient have a friend or relative who can assist? _____

Health Habits and Lifestyle

1. Smoking:

   Smokes cigarettes ___
   Number smoked per day ___
   Smokes pipe/cigars ___
   Nonsmoker ___
   Quit smoking during the past year ___

2. Physical activity (include any activity on the job)

	Minutes/day	Times/week
Walking	_____	_____
Jogging	_____	_____
Swimming	_____	_____
Bicycling	_____	_____
Other:	_____	_____

   Specify _____

3. Does patient seem to be a time-oriented, stressed, or very structured person?

   Yes ___   No ___

4. Has the patient had any severe personal problems in the past 12 months? (For example, death of a family member, marital problems, divorce, lawsuits, job change, serious problems with children, accidents, or evidence of alcohol or drug abuse?)

5. Will family members support the need for changing food habits? Yes ___ No ___

Comments:

_____

_____

_____

_____

_____

_____

In addition to the health history data described above, it is useful to ask for the age of onset of the patient's obesity and changes in weight in adulthood. Understanding the patient's weight history will help the nurse assist the patient in setting realistic weight loss goals.

If obesity began in childhood, it may be harder to treat (Pemberton, 1987). In this case, more modest weight loss goals or prevention of further weight gain may be appropriate. If obesity began in adult life, it may be associated with greater health risks. If the patient has lost and re-gained weight with previous dieting attempts, permanent changes in eating and lifestyle behavior must be stressed.

Physical Examination

Once the nurse has obtained all the background possible, he or she can turn to the patient's physical appearance for clues to nutritional status.

PHYSICAL SIGNS

General appearance:

Good nutrition: Alert, responsive, energetic, good endurance, sleeps well, vigorous

Poor nutrition: Listless, apathetic, cachexia, easily fatigued, no energy, falls asleep easily, looks tired, apathetic

Weight:

Good nutrition: Weight normal for height, age, and body build

Poor nutrition: Overweight or underweight

Posture:

Good nutrition: Erect posture, arms and legs straight

Poor nutrition: Sagging shoulders, sunken chest, humped back

Muscles:

Good nutrition: Well developed, firm, good tone, some fat under skin

Poor nutrition: Flaccid, poor tone, underdeveloped, tender, "wasted" appearance, cannot walk properly

Nervous system:

Good nutrition: Good attention span, not irritable or restless, normal reflexes, psychological stability

Poor nutrition: Inattentive, irritable, confused, paresthesias, loss of position and vibratory sense, weakness and tenderness of muscles, decreased or lost ankle and knee reflexes

Gastrointestinal function:

Good nutrition: Good appetite and digestion, normal regular elimination, no palpable organs or masses

Poor nutrition: Anorexia, indigestion, constipation or diarrhea, liver or spleen enlargement

Cardiovascular function:

Good nutrition: Normal heart rate and rhythm, no murmurs, blood pressure normal for age

Poor nutrition: Rapid heart rate (above 100 beats per minute), enlarged heart, abnormal rhythm, elevated blood pressure

Hair:

Good nutrition: Shiny, lustrous, firm, not easily pulled out, healthy scalp

Poor nutrition: Stringy, dull, brittle, dry, thin and sparse, depigmented, can be easily pulled out

Overall skin condition:

Good nutrition: Smooth, slightly moist, good color

Poor nutrition: Rough, dry, scaly, pale, pigmented, irritated, bruises, petechiae

Face and neck:

Good nutrition: Skin color uniform, smooth, pink, with a healthy appearance and not swollen

Poor nutrition: Greasy, discolored, scaly, swollen, dark skin over cheeks and under eyes, lumpiness or flakiness of skin around nose and mouth

Lips:

Good nutrition: smooth, good color, moist, not chapped or swollen

Poor nutrition: Dry, scaly, swollen, redness and swelling (cheilosis) or angular lesions at corners of the mouth or fissures or scars (stomatitis)

Mouth, oral membranes:

Good nutrition: Reddish pink mucous membranes in oral cavity

Poor nutrition: Swollen, boggy oral mucous membranes

Gums:

Good nutrition: Good pink color, healthy, red, no swelling or bleeding

Poor nutrition: Spongy, bleed easily, marginal redness, inflamed, gums receding

Tongue:

Good nutrition: Good pink color or deep reddish in appearance, not swollen or smooth, surface papillae present, no lesion

Poor nutrition: Swelling, scarlet and raw, magenta color, glossitis, hyperemic and hypertrophic papillae, atrophic papillae

Teeth:

Good nutrition: No cavities, no pain, bright, straight, no crowding, well-shaped jaw, clean, no discoloration

Poor nutrition: Unfilled cavities, absent teeth, worn surfaces, mottled (fluorosis), malpositioned

Eyes:

Good nutrition: Bright, clear, shiny, no sores at corners of eyelids, membranes moist and a healthy pink color, no prominent blood vessels or mount of tissue or sclera, no fatigue circles underneath eyes

Poor nutrition: Pale conjunctivas, conjunctival injection, dryness, signs of infection, Bitot's spots, redness and fissuring of eyelid corners, dryness of eye membrane, dull appearance of cornea (corneal xerosis), soft cornea (keratomalacia)

Neck:

Good nutrition: No enlargement of glands

Poor nutrition: Thyroid enlarged

Nails:

Good nutrition: Firm, pink

Poor nutrition: Brittle, ridged, spoon-shaped

Legs, feet:

Good nutrition: No tenderness, weakness, or swelling, good color

Poor nutrition: Edema, tender calf, tingling weakness

Skeleton:

Good nutrition: No malformations

Poor nutrition: Bowlegs, knock-knees, chest deformity at diaphragm, beaded ribs, prominent scapulas

ANTHROPOMETRIC ASSESSMENT

Weight for Height Tables

Standard weight and height tables similar to the Metropolitan Life Insurance Company tables first appeared in Europe in 1836. In later years the life insurance industry developed tables as a guide for evaluating life insurance applicants. Insurance industry standards were established on the basis that overweight people were poor insurance risks. As a result these people had to pay higher premiums, if they were offered coverage at all.

In March 1983, the Metropolitan Life Insurance Company issued its "new" and adjusted weight ranges for men and women, based on data for 4.2 million persons over 22 years (See Table 4.1).

Table 4.1 HEIGHT–WEIGHT TABLES FOR ADULTS (1983)

These tables are based on a weight-height mortality study conducted by the Society of Actuaries and the Association of Life Insurance Directors of America, Metropolitan Life Insurance Company, revised 1983.

Women

Height Ft. In.		Frame* Small	Medium	Large
4	10	102-111	109-121	118-131
4	11	103-113	111-123	120-134
5	0	104-115	113-126	122-137
5	1	106-118	115-129	125-140
5	2	108-121	118-132	128-143
5	3	111-124	121-135	131-147
5	4	114-127	124-138	134-151
5	5	117-130	127-141	137-155
5	6	120-133	130-144	140-159
5	7	123-136	133-147	143-163
5	8	126-139	136-150	146-167
5	9	129-142	139-153	149-170
5	10	132-145	142-156	152-173
5	11	135-148	145-159	155-176
6	0	138-151	148-162	158-179

Men

Height Ft. In.		Frame* Small	Medium	Large
5	2	128-134	131-141	138-150
5	3	130-136	133-143	140-153
5	4	132-138	135-145	142-156
5	5	134-140	137-148	144-160
5	6	136-142	139-151	146-164
5	7	138-145	142-154	149-168
5	8	140-148	145-157	152-172
5	9	142-151	148-160	155-176
5	10	144-154	151-163	158-180
5	11	146-157	154-166	161-184
6	0	149-160	157-170	164-188
6	1	152-164	160-174	168-192
6	2	155-168	164-178	172-197
6	3	158-172	167-182	176-202
6	4	162-176	171-187	181-207

* — Weights at ages 25 to 50, based on lowest mortality. Height includes 1-inch heels. Weight for women includes 3 lb. for indoor clothing. Weight for men includes 5 lb. for indoor clothing.

Despite the fact that tables such as these are widely used to establish so-called ideal weights, there is controversy about their use. During the past few years, researchers and nutritionists have questioned the use of such tables and the philosophy behind them. Even Metropolitan Life has dropped the words "ideal" and "desirable" from their height and weight tables. One of the problems was that people with the lowest mortality rates tended to weigh less than the weight ranges given. Also, insurance policyholders aren't representative of the population at large, for at least three reasons: (1) Policyholders are largely white, middle-class adult males; (2) underwriting practices vary widely, from strict to lenient, and since weight measurements and health data can be inaccurate, self-disclosed, or sometimes even falsely reported, they are unsuitable for public health purposes; (3) finally, the population of American policyholders doesn't reflect the general population and its incidence of chronic disease or acute illnesses because such people usually do not apply for insurance or may be rejected if they do. Also, overweight persons charged higher rates may have been motivated to buy health insurance from fears of a hidden health problem that could lead to early death.

Of course, no one weight is right for all people of the same height and sex. Some individuals have large frames. Others are delicate. Still others fall in between. The example of the well-muscled football player comes to mind again. Although his ideal weight may be 170 pounds according to tables like the one above, he might weigh 225 due to extremely well-developed muscles. A woman may have an ideal weight of 120 pounds but may weigh 140 pounds, yet not have any excess fat.

Other groups feel that the average weights are too high. In the Duke University Program, weights for men and women are a great deal lower than the Metropolitan Life weights. The standards set at Duke are that a woman's goal weight should be 100 pounds for the first 5 feet of height, then five pounds for every inch over that. For men, 106 pounds are allotted for the first 5 feet, then six pounds for every inch thereafter. Thus, a woman 5' 4" tall would have an ideal weight of 120 pounds, rather than 124-128 pounds. An average man who is 5' 11" would have an ideal weight of 172 pounds, instead of 154-166 pounds.

Reuban Andres (1985), clinical director of the Gerontology Research Center at the National Institute on Aging, was one of the first persons to be concerned about excess thinness and the effects of moderate overweight on older persons. He noted that the Metropolitan Life tables were too restrictive for older persons and too liberal for young adults. Instead, he suggests using the following formula for finding a "safe" weight range for older patients. Older people can also do this themselves, to find their own best weight.

1. Measure your patient's height without shoes, in inches, and divide this figure by 66.

2. Multiply this result by itself.

3. Multiply that result by patient's age, plus 100.

The resulting number is the middle of a "safe" weight range. This weight is usually within about 15 pounds in either direction, unless hypertension or diabetes is present.

Because most persons have a progressive increase in percentage of body fat as they get older, the safe range of weight rises with age. Older people who gain about 8 to 10 pounds per decade may actually be helping themselves stay healthier. Unless hypertension or diabetes is a factor, the added weight may have a protective effect in older age (Simonson, 1983).

Most height-weight tables are set up to include variations depending on body frame, or relative size of bones. This is also a controversial area, and some scientists feel that frame types were created simply by dividing the weight distribution of all the life insurance data into thirds and labeling those thirds "small," "medium," and "large." Even the American Medical Association has pointed out the difficulties of determining frame size. For others, however, it at least gives one more variable to help determine appropriate weight.

Dr. Simonson (1983) suggests the following method for estimating frame type:

1. Measure your height to the nearest quarter of an inch. Have a friend or your spouse measure the circumference of your shoulders with a tape measure. Add the two figures. If the total of the two measurements is less than 99 inches, you have a "small frame." If the total is 99.1 to 106.0 inches, you have a "medium" frame. If the total is more than 106 inches, you have a "large" or "big-boned" frame.

2. Measure the circumference of the wrist on your dominant hand. For women, a wrist measurement less than 6 inches indicates a small frame; 6 to 6 1/2 inches, a medium frame; and over 6 1/2 inches, a large frame. For men, a wrist measurement less than 6 inches indicates a small frame, 6 to 7 inches, a medium frame, and more than 7 inches, a large frame.

Dr. Simonson has another method to check out ideal weight, once frame size is apparent.

For men: Multiply height in stocking feet by 4. Subtract 128 from the total. This number forms the ideal weight if the man is medium-boned. If a man is small-boned, he should subtract 10 percent from this total. If he is large-boned, he should add 10 percent.

Example: A large-boned man who is 73 inches tall multiplies 73 times 4, getting 292. He subtracts 128 to get 164; then adds 10 percent (because of large frame), or 16.4, to get an ideal weight of 180.4 pounds.

For women: Women multiply their height in inches by 3.5, then subtract 108 from the total. They subtract another 10 percent for small bones, or add 10 percent for large bones.

Example: A medium-boned woman who is 66 inches tall multiplies 66 times 3.5, for a total of 231. She then subtracts 108, to get an ideal weight of 123.0 pounds.

Relative Weight

The term *relative weight* expresses a patient's weight in pounds as a percentage of desirable body weight as defined in weight for height tables, usually the Metropolitan Life Insurance Tables. Relative weight is calculated by dividing current weight in pounds by the midpoint of the desirable weight range for individuals with a medium frame.

Consider, for example, a women who is 5' 8" tall and weighs 165 pounds. Using the 1983 Height-Weight Tables for Adults from the previous section, the midpoint of the medium-frame weight range for this height is 143 pounds. Thus:

$$165 \text{ pounds} \div 143 \text{ pounds} \times 100 = 115 \text{ percent}$$

Generally, a relative body weight of 120 percent is considered overweight, while a relative body weight of 130 percent of more is considered obese.

Body Mass Index

Because of the limitations of weight for height tables as discussed earlier, body weight is often described in terms of *body mass index* (BMI, also called Quetelet's index). This index is not only useful for relating body weight to height, but is also helpful for evaluating the percentage of body fat.

Table 4.2 BMI: Normal Age-adjusted Levels

Age range (yr.)	BMI (kg/m^2)
19–24	19–24
25–34	20–25
35–44	21–26
45–54	21–26
55–64	23–28
65+	24–29

Table 4.3 BMI and Degree of Obesity

Degree of Obesity	BMI
Desirable weight	21–22
Overweight	25
Obesity	30
Medically significant obesity	35
Super obesity	40
Morbid obesity	45
Super morbid obesity	≥ 50

Source: National Institute of Health Technology Assessment Conference, 1992. *Annals of Internal Medicine*

The formula for the BMI (Quetelet index) divides the weight by the height squared. The BMI is calculated by dividing the body weight (in kilograms) by the square of the height (in meters), or BMI= kg/m^2. [A simplified version of this formula is W(weight)/ H(height)^2.]

The BMI has the best correlation with body fat, and thus may be a preferable way to measure overweight and obesity. Table 4.2 gives recommendations for levels of the BMI, adjusted for age. The adjustment for age was devised after studies by Andres (1985) showed that age-adjustment of weight is important. He calculated the BMI at which minimum mortality occurred for both men and women at each decade during life. Data for men and women rise with age and there is no difference according to sex.

An overweight person could be defined as having a BMI from the top of the normal range to less than 5 kg/m2 above normal for age or body weight between the upper limit of normal and 20 percent above that limit. An obese person would have a BMI greater than 5 kg/m2 above the upper limit of normal, triceps plus subscapular skinfold of 45 mm (males) and 69 mm (females), body weight more than 20 percent above the upper limit for height, or body fat 25 percent in males or 30 percent in females.

Blackburn (1987) defines degrees of obesity using BMI in another way as shown in Table 4.3.

One disadvantage of using BMI is that people have difficulty thinking in terms of ratios and how they translate into pounds. Table 4.4 shows how BMI relates to weight for height and provides a useful reference for determining BMI of patients.

Fat Distribution

In addition to relative weight or BMI, nurses should also assess body fat distribution, specifically upper body versus lower body. Men tend to accumulate fat more in the abdominal area, or upper body, while women tend to accumulate fat more in the hip region, or lower body. Upper body obesity is associated with greater health risks than lower body obesity.

The ratio of waist circumference to hip circumference provides an objective estimate of body fat distribution. Waist to hip ratios greater than 1.0 for men and greater than 0.8 for women indicate greater risk for cardiovascular disease and diabetes (Surgeon General's Report on Nutrition and Health, 1988).

Table 4.4 Body Weights in Pounds According to Height and Body Mass Index*

| | Body Mass Index (kg/m²) | | | | | | | | | | | | | |
Height (in.)	19	20	21	22	23	24	25	26	27	28	29	30	35	40
						Body Weight (lb.)								
58	91	96	100	105	110	115	119	124	129	134	138	143	167	191
59	94	99	104	109	114	119	124	128	133	138	143	148	173	198
60	97	102	107	112	118	123	128	133	138	143	148	153	179	204
61	100	106	111	116	122	127	132	137	143	148	153	158	185	211
62	104	109	115	120	126	131	136	142	147	153	158	164	191	218
63	107	113	118	124	130	135	141	146	152	158	163	169	197	225
64	110	116	122	128	134	140	145	151	157	163	169	174	204	232
65	114	120	126	132	138	144	150	156	162	168	174	180	210	240
66	118	124	130	136	142	148	155	161	167	173	179	186	216	247
67	121	127	134	140	146	153	159	166	172	178	185	191	223	255
68	125	131	138	144	151	158	164	171	177	184	190	197	230	262
69	128	135	142	149	155	162	169	176	182	189	196	203	236	270
70	132	139	146	153	160	167	174	181	188	195	202	207	243	278
71	136	143	150	157	165	172	179	186	193	200	208	215	250	286
72	140	147	154	162	169	177	184	191	199	206	213	221	258	294
73	144	151	159	166	174	182	189	197	204	212	219	227	265	302
74	148	155	163	171	179	186	194	202	210	218	225	233	272	311
75	152	160	168	176	184	192	200	208	216	224	232	240	279	319
76	156	164	172	180	189	197	205	213	221	230	238	246	287	328

*Each entry gives the body weight in pounds (lb.) for a person of a given height and body mass index. Pounds have been rounded off. To use the table, find the appropriate height in the left-hand column. Move across the row to a given weight. The number at the top of the column is the body mass index for the height and weight.

Source: G. A. Bray and D. S. Gray. "Obesity. Part 1 Pathogenisis." Reprinted by permission of *The Western Journal of Medicine*, 1988: 149: 429–441.

Body Composition

Precise determination of body fat content requires sophisticated methods such as underwater weighing, radiographic analysis, electrical impedance, or ultrasound techniques. Since most of these are not practical for use in clinical settings, anthropometric measurements can be used to estimate body fat content. Besides weight for height, BMI, and waist to hip ratio, careful measurements of skinfold thickness can also provide useful estimates of body fat content.

Most hospitals and clinics use standard millimeter skinfold calipers such as the Lange, Harpenden, or Holtain type. The sum of skinfolds taken at more than one site provides a more accurate estimate of body fat. For men, chest, abdomen, and thigh skinfolds are often used. For women, triceps and suprailium (just above the crest of the hip bone) are often used. Subscapular skinfold thicknesses are also frequently measured.

Several groups have devised equations to predict body fat from skinfold thicknesses taken at various sites. However, these equations usually apply to a specific population and have not been standardized for broad use.

PSYCHOSOCIAL ASSESSMENT

Many obese people overeat in response to psychological and social cues rather than hunger. The three "C's" often describe why people overeat—to *comfort*, to *control*, or to *cope*.

Psychosocial assessment helps clarify the role of food and body weight in the patient's life. Grommet (1988) describes areas that should be explored to assess the obese patient:

1. Experience with past weight loss attempts, weight change, how long weight was maintained, when the program was stopped, and if any problems were encountered.

2. Reasons for wanting to lose weight at this time.

3. Whether the patient thinks this weight loss attempt will differ from any previous attempts.

4. Are there significant life events that may have caused weight gain?

5. Has the patient experienced any lifestyle changes that might make weight loss more difficult?

6. How do family members feel about the patient's obesity and desire to lose weight?

7. Do specific moods of the patient influence amount of food eaten or physical activity?

DIETARY ASSESSMENT

Dietary assessment should reveal usual eating patterns, types and quantities of foods eaten, and information about the eating environment such as food-related thoughts and eating cues. A registered dietitian will often be responsible for dietary assessment of the obese patient. A careful history of diet and nutritional information in relation to the patient's living situation and other personal, psychosocial, and economic problems, is another essential part of the nutritional assessment of any patient. It isn't always easy to get accurate information because most overweight persons, just like everyone else, aren't really aware of everything they are eating. Most people have no idea how many calories they consume during an average day, and many fool themselves into thinking they are being careful and cutting back, not taking into account the late-night refrigerator raids.

Food Records

A food record (also called a diet diary) kept for 24 hours or longer can give patients and their health care professionals a better idea of actual food consumption. A diet diary, kept for 24 hours or longer, can give a clearer picture of what they're really eating. Having a patient monitor his or her eating habits will accomplish three things: It will help the patient (1) become aware of his own behavior, such as eating too much late at night; (2) set goals for change, for example, substituting lower-calorie snacks for heavy dinners; and (3) find ways to reinforce or support the new behavior (Simonson, 1983). Many weight-loss groups ask participants to keep an honest and detailed food diary during much of the program.

Awareness of food problems begins with the patient's participation in the first assessment. It continues with the patient learning to observe his own behavior throughout the counseling period and keeping records.

Record-keeping or self-monitoring by the patient can be an important way to help him achieve long-term behavioral changes. A detailed food diary is very useful at the beginning, and at differing times throughout the diet. In some cases, it is helpful to have a prospective patient keep a three-day food diary before he or she comes in the first time.

Why keep a food diary? Self-monitoring can help the patient in many ways:

1. It can provide information about eating habits and the factors that influence them.

2. It helps the patient get involved in observing and analyzing his own diet habits.

3. It increases the patient's awareness of his diet and behavior.

4. It gives the health practitioner and patient something to review objectively and impartially — they can focus on problems on the record, not on the patient.

5. It reinforces new behavior, and serves as a reminder that allows the individual to make corrections. For example, a patient may find he is consuming too many high-calorie beverages, so he may decide to switch to sugar-free iced tea, colas, coffee, or water.

6. It increases the patient's skill in manipulating the diet to achieve desired results. For example, the patient may find a variety of low-fat animal and vegetable protein sources, or find acceptable snack foods that fit into the daily food pattern.

7. It increases interaction between the health practitioner and patient.

When counseling a patient, it is essential to know the patient's usual diet pattern. Having the patient keep a three-day food diary (some use a week-long, or even a 14-day form), provides a baseline for planning and measuring later changes.

Be sure to have a well-designed form ready at the first meeting, and ask the patient to start keeping records soon afterwards. Depending on what is being assessed, the diary may include types and amounts of food eaten, the location, time of day, time spent eating, what else the patient was doing at the same time, such as watching television or reading. Was the patient with anyone, and what was the overall mood at the time of eating?

The diary can have many forms, including exercise data. It should include most of the following information:

1. Type of day — workday or non-workday
2. Place food was eaten and the circumstances — at home or away, during a party, in a restaurant, etc.
3. The kind of food eaten
4. The time food was eaten
5. The amount eaten, as accurately as possible
6. How the food was prepared

Some also include suggestions to patients for completing food records. The following are suggested by the NIH (1987):

1. Records should include all meals any time of the day or night, snacks, coffee breaks, soft drink breaks, cocktails, beer, anything you nibble, every refrigerator raid.

2. Try to write down any foods immediately in the food record.

The following questions are particularly important in regard to high-fat foods or cholesterol-containing foods:

3. Were fats or oils used in cooking or baking? If so, what brands were used?

4. Did you use salad dressings or mayonnaise in salads or on sandwiches?

5. Did you add fat to vegetables while cooking or afterward? If so, what kind did you add?

6. What kind of milk did you drink or use in cooking?

7. Did you eat margarine or butter on bread, toast, sandwiches, rolls, potatoes, etc.? If you used margarine, what brand did you choose?

8. Were gravies, sauces, or syrups added to any of your foods?

9. What cuts of meat were eaten? Did you trim off the fat or not?

10. What ingredients were used in mixed dishes, sandwiches, etc.?

11. Record in ounces all beverages, including alcoholic beverages.

12. Be sure to include how many and what size bread, rolls, crackers, raw fruits and vegetables, cookies, candies, snack items, etc.

13. Record by servings and size: pie, cake, coffee cake

14. Record in cups or by servings: potatoes, rice, fruits, vegetables, cereals, soups, casseroles.

15. Record in teaspoons or tablespoons any jellies, jams, sugar, syrup, sauces, gravies, salad dressings, butter, margarine, nuts, and seeds.

Some programs also include a snack record form that the patient can carry in pocket or purse, to record foods eaten away from home. This record should also include the day, the time of day, whether the food was eaten while the person was alone or with someone (list the person), the type of food eaten, and the amount eaten.

Accuracy is important. It is vital to emphasize to the patient that accuracy is important. Select methods that are easy to use, convenient, and readily available when the behavior occurs. Some encourage the patient to make suggestions on what to record as well as how to do so. For example, the patient may find it easier to carry a pocket-sized food diary with her at all times, or attach a "breakfast record" to the refrigerator, or keep a list of evening snacks on the dresser.

Keep instructions clear. Make sure the patient understands the purpose of keeping the food diary. Also, go over any form or any part of the form that might be confusing, or, if in doubt, have the patient fill out a sample page. If asked to record amounts of food, make sure the patient knows how to estimate amounts of food, and has a good food scale and measuring cups and spoons at home. Use familiar household measurements with cups and spoons or food models, to relate portions to familiar shapes and sizes. It's good to be specific about sizes and portions; an apple, for example, may be small or so large it takes two hands to hold it—quite a difference in calories!

Be sure the records the patient is keeping are relevant to the dietary problem at hand. Don't ask for more information than needed, and stress that the patient need only keep records if the information is useful.

Encourage the patient to make prompt notations about eating. Nothing is more frustrating than trying to remember what one had for lunch when it's dinnertime.

Use the records to observe patterns, not to judge behavior. Avoid expressing disapproval. Remember, many people are reluctant to reveal their full eating habits, especially if they seem embarrassing or unhealthy. Not many persons want to admit eating a half-gallon of rocky road ice cream or two tubs of popcorn, or fasting one day to gorge the next. Instead, whatever the eating habits may be, the purpose of the diary is to help both nurse and patient accurately assess the patient's current diet, plan changes, and identify problem eating behaviors. Records are only an aid, not a judgment. The records should be as complete as possible, and should include even tiny portions of food, such as half a tablespoonful, or just a bite. It all adds up.

The diet diary may reveal some surprising things. A person who feels she is eating like a bird may actually be tasting and sampling food, all day long, and eating far more calories than she would if she ate three moderate meals. Or a man who eats a light breakfast and lunch may be defeating himself by eating a calorie-laden dinner and snacking steadily into the late-evening hours.

For food records to be useful and accurate, patients must pay careful attention to estimating portion size. To increase accuracy, the health professional can ask patients to weigh and measure foods for a few days or anytime they are unsure of portion sizes. A recent study by Lichtman and colleagues (1992) found that some obese subjects who reported difficulty losing weight on a low calorie diet under-reported calorie intake by almost 50 percent.

It is important to use the information gained from a patient's food diaries, especially if he or she has faithfully kept a diary. By reviewing the records together, health professionals can teach patients about foods that are high in cholesterol or fat. These records can also show the patient's problem areas; for example, extra-large portions of high-fat foods, or lack of vegetables.

A food diary can be invaluable for patients because it allows them to use self-monitoring, an important means of continuing to assess the diet and measure change. Encouraging the patient to be involved in assessment and self-observation is a good strategy of beginning, promoting, and helping him adhere to the diet.

According to nutritionists at the NIH, self-monitoring tends to change behavior through the development of an increased awareness of self, and tends to do this in a favorable direction. Self-monitoring also has an important second benefit: It serves as a reminder which allows the patient to take self-corrective action.

Twenty-four Hour Food Recall

For some patients, keeping records simply is not feasible. Some persons aren't willing to take the time needed to fill out a regular diet diary. Others are unable to do so because of language difficulties or problems with reading and writing. There are other ways to get the information, such as having the patient call in on a regular basis to give a 24-hour recall of foods eaten, or asking the patient to complete a food checklist (see below), or simply continuing to ask pertinent questions about how well he is doing if he is trying to change certain diet patterns.

To take a 24-hour food recall, the interviewer asks the patient to recall everything he or she ate and drank for the previous day. For persons working odd hours or eating at night, it is important to include a complete 24-hour period starting at 12:00 a.m. To help the patient remember what was eaten and drunk, ask what he or she did that day. For instance, the beginning of a 24-hour recall interview might proceed as follows:

> "About what time did you get up yesterday? And what was the first thing you ate or drank? Then what did you do? Did you eat or drink anything then?"

Some patients might have an easier time remembering what they ate and drank from the most recent meal backwards:

> "Did you eat or drink anything in the middle of the night last night? Did you have anything before you went to bed? What did you have for supper?"

The interviewer must remember to ask specific questions about portion size; how food was prepared; and whether toppings such as butter, margarine, or dressing were added at the table. Food models can often assist patients in estimating portion size.

Twenty-four hour recalls are fairly quick, inexpensive, and do not require a high level of patient effort. Interactive computerized 24-hour recall programs are also available. However, food intake in one 24-hour period may not give a true representation of usual food intake. For more accurate estimates of usual intake, several recalls are needed. Some patients may have trouble remembering what they ate the previous day, hence, underestimating food intake. Also, some individuals tend to tailor recall to what they think the interviewer expects to hear.

Food Frequency Questionnaires

Questionnaires that ask how frequently the patient consumes certain foods can also give insight into dietary habits of obese persons. Food frequency questionnaires are quick and easy to complete and provide insight on consumption of certain types of high-calorie or high-fat foods. However, food frequency questionnaires do not provide very accurate information on quantity.

Following is a sample questionnaire that combines weight history and lifestyle habits with food frequency questions:

1. What has been your heaviest weight?

2. How much did you weigh at the following ages: birth, age 10, age 15, age 25, and now?

3. Describe the following members of your family as thin, average, heavy, or obese: your spouse, yourself, your mother, your father, your sisters, your brothers, your own children.

4. How do you spend a typical day? Ask the patient to elaborate, for example, reading, studying, watching television (remember the earlier figures about the average child spending nearly 23 hours a week in front of the television?), or physical activities, such as aerobics, jogging, or traveling.

5. What type of job do you have — how do you spend a typical day on the job?

6. Do you eat out often? How frequently?

7. Do you have any sleeping problems? How many hours do you sleep during an average night?

8. How much exercise do you get regularly? Are you less active than you once were?

9. What are your interests and hobbies?

10. Do you have long stretches of time with nothing to do? If so, can you explain why?

11. What are the reasons you want to lose weight?

12. Why do you think you are overweight?

13. How much do you want to lose, and what do you think is your goal weight?

14. Have you ever devised a diet of your own? Describe it, and how long you were on it.

15. How many times have you tried to lose weight in the past? What ways did you use? Did they work, or did you regain your lost weight?

16. When do you usually eat your meals? Breakfast? Lunch? Dinner?

17. Do you eat vegetables every day? Fruits?

18. Do you eat cereals and whole grains?

19. Do you drink milk or eat dairy products? How often?

20. How many cups of coffee and/or tea do you drink every day?

21. Do you drink soft drinks, and, if so, how many per day?

22. Do you drink alcoholic beverages? How much? How often?

23. Estimate your total fluid intake per day. Would you estimate this to be 1 quart? 2 quarts? Less?

24. Do you ever estimate your daily caloric intake, and can you do it correctly? If so, what is the average day's total calories for you?

25. Are there types of foods you like better than others; are there types you dislike more than others?

26. How many meals per day do you eat?

27. How often do you eat snacks?

28. What do you eat during snack time?

29. What makes you choose the foods you do? Environment? Hunger? Stress? Taste, sight of food, craving for a certain food? Social pressure? Time pressure? Travel? Ethnic or cultural conditioning? Habit?

30. Do you have specific associations with certain foods? (That is, do certain foods evoke emotions or association with persons or places?)

ANOREXIA NERVOSA AND BULIMIA

Health professionals who assess individuals desiring to lose weight may also encounter individuals with bulimia, anorexia nervosa, or both. Both conditions are fairly common eating disorders and are recognized as serious psychiatric disorders with sometimes severe physical complications (National Research Council, 1989). Nurses should be aware of diagnostic criteria of these disorders and make the appropriate referral.

Anorexia nervosa occurs most commonly in adolescent girls and is characterized by extreme weight loss, disturbances in body image, and an intense fear of becoming overweight. As many as one in 100 females between 12 and 18 years of age have anorexia (Farley, 1992). Diagnostic criteria for anorexia nervosa include:

- Refusal to maintain weight above the lowest weight considered normal for height and age,
- Fear of becoming obese, even though patient is underweight,
- Distorted body image, and
- In non-pregnant women, missing three consecutive menstrual periods (Farley, 1992).

In contrast to anorexia, bulimia affects a much greater portion of the population, but, especially young females. Some studies indicate that up to 18 percent of college-age women are bulimic (Farley, 1992). Bulimia is characterized by episodes of binge eating followed by purging (i.e., self-induced vomit-

ing, fasting, use of laxatives or diuretics). Bulimia can be difficult to diagnose and treat. Individuals suffering from bulimia usually have normal or slightly higher than normal body weights.

Diagnostic criteria for bulimia include:

- Recurrent binge eating averaging at least two episodes a week for at least three months (some binges can be several thousand calories at a time),
- Lack of control over eating during binges,
- Regular purging through self-induced vomiting, use of laxatives, diuretics, strict dieting, fasting, or vigorous exercise, and
- Obsession with body shape and weight.

In addition to anorexia nervosa and bulimia, compulsive binge eating without purging may affect a high portion of obese individuals. DeZwaan and colleagues (1992) found that 34 percent of obese females in a controlled weight-reduction program had recurrent episodes of binge eating. Binge eating often complicates obesity intervention, and binge eaters are more likely to drop out of programs than non-binge eaters. Individuals with compulsive eating disorders should receive psychotherapy to address the underlying issues causing the compulsion.

Comprehensive medical, anthropometric, psychosocial and dietary assessment provide important baseline data for designing effective treatment strategies. The next chapter discusses the most common approaches to obesity treatment and their indications for use.

EXAM QUESTIONS

Chapter 4

Questions 30-39

30. Which of the following is least relevant in obtaining a health history from an obese individual?

    a. the patient's weight at birth
    b. age of onset of the patient's obesity
    c. experience with previous weight loss attempts
    d. incidence of obesity in mother or father

31. Which of the following can be a physical sign of poor nutrition?

    a. smooth, slightly moist skin
    b. psychological stability
    c. reddish pink mucous membranes in oral cavity
    d. dry, thin hair

32. Which of the following is a healthy level for body mass index?

    a. 15
    b. 21
    c. 35
    d. 50

33. Why is an ideal-weight chart, such as that published by Metropolitan Life Insurance Company, not the best weight guide?

    a. It is devised from data taken from a large sample of policyholders.
    b. Health data are too old to be accurate.
    c. The policyholders are mostly older individuals.
    d. The policyholders are mostly white, male and from middle-class groups.

34. How is a "safe" weight range for older people calculated?

    a. by height, weight, and ideal-weight charts
    b. height (in inches) divided by 66, times itself, times age, plus 100
    c. by studying mortality tables
    d. height (in meters) squared, divided by 30 times weight (in kilograms)

35. How is the body mass index (BMI) calculated?

    a. by dividing the weight (in kilograms) by the height (in meters) squared
    b. by evaluating the percentage of body fat
    c. by subtracting the weight from the height
    d. by dividing the weight (in pounds) by the height (in inches) squared

36. The term *relative weight* refers to:

    a. current weight in pounds divided by the midpoint of desirable weight range, times 100
    b. weight history of the patient's relatives
    c. another term for body mass index
    d. midpoint of desirable weight range

37. How is the waist-to-hip ratio used?

    a. to detect diabetes mellitus or stroke
    b. as a measure of body fat distribution
    c. to assure that surgical gowns fit properly
    d. to predict body weight changes

38. Which of the following techniques is not used in dietary assessment of obese individuals?

    a. food lists
    b. food records
    c. food recalls
    d. food frequency questionnaires

39. Which of the following is a symptom of bulimia?

    a. refusal to maintain weight above the lowest weight considered normal for height and age
    b. for non-pregnant women, missing three consecutive menstrual periods
    c. regular purging through self-induced vomiting, use of laxatives, diuretics, strict dieting or exercise
    d. distorted body image

CHAPTER 5

PLANNING
WEIGHT MANAGEMENT OPTIONS

CHAPTER OBJECTIVE

After reading this chapter, you will be able to indicate appropriate weight management choices for patients with different degrees of obesity and medical risk.

LEARNING OBJECTIVES

After studying this chapter, you will be able to:

1. Identify the features of balanced low-calorie diets, very low-calorie diets, and behavior modification techniques.

2. Discuss the effects of pharmacological and surgical interventions on weight loss.

3. Specify conditions for which weight loss is contraindicated.

INTRODUCTION

Four recent national surveys have asked respondents questions about weight loss (National Institutes of Health, 1992). Among women, 84 percent of those trying to lose weight had cut back their calories, and 60 to 63 percent were trying to exercise more. Among men, 76 to 78 percent had cut back their calories, and 60 to 62 percent were trying to exercise more. Among students, methods to lose weight (from most to least frequently used) included exercise, skipping meals, diet pills, and self-induced vomiting. Clearly, education is needed on appropriate methods of weight loss.

In the simplest form, weight loss principles can be summarized by the calories in–calories out equation. Just as weight gain occurs when calories taken in chronically exceed calories expended, weight loss is accomplished when calories taken in are less than calories expended. Long-term weight maintenance is achieved by balancing calories in with calories out. But just as there are many causes of obesity, there are also many ways to treat the disease. No one approach works for everyone.

ELEMENTS OF SUCCESS

According to Robison (1993), successful weight control programs:

1. Are individualized to the needs and medical status of the patient.

2. Are multi-disciplinary in nature, involving trained practitioners from medicine, psychology, nutrition, and exercise physiology all working as a team with the patient.

3. Are long-term, with on-going intervention and support even after weight loss has been accomplished.

4. Address psychological and social barriers to lifetime weight control.

5. Encourage family and peer support.

6. Foster positive self-image and better quality of life.

Regardless of the means to accomplish weight loss, weight loss interventions should emphasize lifetime changes in diet, exercise, and behavior to promote permanent weight control. Aggressive weight loss interventions should only be undertaken with comprehensive medical screening and supervision.

SETTING REALISTIC GOALS

Setting realistic goals is another element of successful weight loss intervention. As Dr. Mervyn Willard (1991) of the Texas Tech University Health Sciences Center states, "Weight loss by itself is not a worthwhile treatment goal, because weight is often regained." Rather, maintenance of weight loss must be the ultimate goal of any obesity intervention program. Weight loss requires only a short-term energy deficit. Weight control, however, requires life-long behavior changes.

Achieving this ultimate goal will probably require a series of short-term goals, including goals for weight loss. The need for weight loss should be driven by health considerations, not cosmetic ones. In a national consensus conference on obesity (National Institutes of Health, 1985), weight loss is recommended for persons exceeding desirable weight by 20 percent or more. For individuals with type II diabetes, high blood pressure, or high blood lipid levels, weight reduction may be helpful at lesser degrees of overweight.

Many patients need not, and probably should not, aim for desirable body weight according to height–weight tables as a short-term goal (Blackburn, 1987). Setting unrealistically high goals can be mentally and physically self-defeating.

In a position paper on weight control, The American Dietetic Association (1989) states:

> "Optimal weight is the most favorable weight for an individual as determined by a variety of factors, such as existing health problems (hypertension, diabetes, heart disease), percentage of body fat, location of excess fat in the body, age, sex, heredity, psychological implications, and realistic weight maintenance goals. For some persons, optimal weight will be more or less than the weight allowed by accepted weight for height tables."

Well-known obesity expert Dr. George Blackburn suggests setting a short-term weight loss goal of 10 to 15 percent of current body weight for any single treatment course, which would last six months to one year. A loss of 10 to 15 percent of body weight improves heart function, blood pressure, glucose tolerance, and many other medical conditions in nine out of ten patients. According to Blackburn, after this weight loss has been maintained for a year or more, the patient can strive to reduce body weight another 10 to 15 percent toward a long-term goal of a BMI of less than 30.

CONSERVATIVE AND AGGRESSIVE THERAPIES

As with other diseases, conservative therapies are usually tried before aggressive therapies. Conservative therapies for obesity treatment include a balanced low-calorie diet, exercise, and behavior change. More aggressive therapies may be appropriate when conservative treatment fails or when the degree of obesity or health risk warrant using them (Perri and colleagues, 1992).

Therapies can also be combined or undertaken in a stepped manner. For example, a phase of balanced low-calorie dieting plus behavior modification and exercise can follow a very low-calorie diet phase. All weight loss interventions must teach sound nutrition, behavior change, and exercise for long-term success.

Dr. Albert Stunkard (1992) of the University of Pennsylvania recommends considering obesity management options based on degree of obesity. Mild obesity, which affects about 90 percent of obese individuals, is usually best treated with conservative therapy unless there are medical indications for more aggressive treatment. Moderate obesity, which affects about 9 percent of obese individuals, can be treated with either conservative or aggressive therapy. Severe obesity, which affects less than 10 percent of obese individuals, is usually best treated with aggressive therapies such as surgery or very low-calorie diets.

BALANCED LOW-CALORIE DIETS

Since good nutrition and balanced low-calorie diets are discussed in Chapters 6 and 7, they will be only briefly reviewed here. Dietary restriction is the most commonly used method for weight loss. Low-calorie diets (LCD) usually provide 1,000 to 1,500 calories daily (about 12 to 15 calories per kilograms of body weight) and allow for weight loss of one to two pounds weekly. Calorie intake below 1,000 is not recommended except with close medical supervision, as discussed in the next section on very low-calorie diets. Balanced LCD of 1,000 calories or more are safe for almost everyone and require minimal medical supervision.

Degree of Obesity	Percent over Desirable Weight	Body Mass Index	Options
Mild	20–39%	27–30	conservative treatment
Moderate	40–100%	30–35	conservative treatment or very low-calorie diet
Severe	>100%	>35	very low-calorie diet or surgery

Contrary to the beliefs of some, most individuals will lose weight on an LCD. Lichtman and colleagues (1992) studied individuals who believed they failed to lose weight on less than 1,200 calories daily by evaluating total energy intake and actual energy expenditure in a metabolic ward. In these individuals, failure to lose weight while dieting was due to under-reporting of calorie intake and overestimation of physical activity.

LCD may have an advantage over more severe levels of caloric restriction. Sweeney and colleagues (1993) studied 30 obese women randomly assigned to either severe or moderate energy restriction with and without exercise. Body composition was determined by underwater weighing and energy expenditure was measured by indirect calorimetry. They found that moderate energy restriction produced greater weight loss relative to energy deficit. Other researchers have found that the expenditure needed to lose 1 percent of body weight is lowest using a LCD compared with using a very low-calorie diet (Stunkard, 1993).

There are many types of LCD, and most commercial weight loss programs use an LCD. According to Smoller and colleagues (1988), three elements that should be included in an LCD are: (1) professional evaluation and supervision (2) a sensible balance of food and nutrients and (3) adjunct exercise and behavior therapy. Diets that are flexible, simple, and individually tailored to fit food preferences, eating patterns, and lifestyle are more likely to be successful than rigid, inflexible diets.

VERY LOW-CALORIE DIETS

In contrast to the low-calorie diets, very low-calorie diets (VLCD) are an aggressive approach to obesity treatment. VLCD were first developed to help prevent the dangerous and sometimes lethal loss of lean body mass with total fasting. However, several deaths occurred on VLCD using liquid protein in the mid- to late 1970s (Lantingua, 1980).

In the 1980s very low-calorie diets (VLCD) again became popular as a means of achieving large weight loss over relatively short time periods (Wadden, 1983). The VLCD of the 1980s differed from earlier VLCD in that they provided high-quality protein and adequate amounts of vitamins and minerals.

The VLCD of today usually provides 600 to 800 calories daily, or about 6 to 10 calories per kilogram of body weight (National Institutes of Health, 1992). Initial weight loss on a VLCD is usually rapid owing to sodium and water loss. Thereafter, weight loss on a VLCD can average two to four pounds weekly (Wadden, 1983). Because of the low calorie level, most of the calories from a VLCD come from high-quality protein to help preserve lean body mass. Protein can be provided from food or from a liquid supplement (Perri, 1992).

Food-based VLCD are also called protein-sparing modified fasts (PSMF) and usually provide 1.5 grams of protein per kilogram of ideal body weight. Protein is derived from lean meats, fish, and poultry, supplemented with vitamins, minerals, and electrolytes.

With liquid VLCD, protein is usually derived from a milk- or egg-based powder that is mixed with water and consumed three to five or more times daily. Vitamins, minerals, and electrolytes are sometimes included in the formula or taken separately. A small amount of carbohydrate is also provided to help minimize water loss and electrolyte abnormalities.

VLCD are usually administered in three phases: (1) a preliminary phase of two to four weeks on a LCD to help the body adjust to calorie restriction (2) a VLCD phase lasting up to 12 weeks and (3) a re-feeding and maintenance phase (Perri, 1980).

VLCD are only appropriate for patients with moderate or severe obesity. Contraindications to a VLCD include recent heart disease, stroke, cancer, type I diabetes, liver or renal failure, or severe psychological disorders (Perri, 1992). Side effects of VLCD can include headaches, fatigue, hypotension, constipation, gallbladder disease, and menstrual irregularity (Atkinson, 1989).

VLCD are considered relatively safe when used appropriately. According to Perri (1992), appropriate use includes:

1. Complete medical screening prior to entry in the program;

2. Exclusion of patients with mild obesity or contraindications;

3. Weekly or biweekly medical supervision while on the program and during the re-feeding phase;

4. Limit of 12 weeks on the VLCD;

5. Routine blood tests and electrocardiograms to evaluate electrolyte balance and cardiac functioning; and

6. Instruction and follow-up during the weight maintenance phase.

While VLCD yield impressive weight loss, long-term results are still discouraging. Combining behavior modification with VLCD may improve results slightly.

Wadden and colleagues (1989) studied weight losses five years after initial treatment with either a VLCD, behavior modification, or a combination of both. Initially weight losses were greatest with the combined therapy. At the end of five years, however, the majority of participants from all three treatment groups had regained all the weight initially lost. Only 11 percent of subjects in the VLCD group, 13 percent of subjects in the behavior modification group, and 27 percent of subjects in the combined VLCD plus behavior modification group maintained losses of 11 pounds or more at the five-year follow-up.

BEHAVIOR MODIFICATION

Behavior modification was originally developed on the theory that faulty eating behavior caused overeating and obesity. The goal of earlier programs was to restructure eating environment and eating behavior for permanent weight loss maintenance. However, weight losses on such programs were modest and weight maintenance was no better than with other interventions (Surgeon General's Report on Nutrition and Health, 1988).

Current behavior modification programs have been broadened and now usually include a balanced low-calorie diet and exercise component. Such programs form the basis of many commercial weight loss regimens. Some behavior modification techniques can also be used in combination with other weight loss therapies, such as very low-calorie diets.

Stunkard (1992) has summarized the key elements in five leading behavior modification manuals. These include:

Stimulus Control. Controlling food cues while grocery shopping, during activities, and at social events; pre-planning and reordering eating environment.

Eating Behavior. Putting utensils down in between bites, chewing slowly, preparing one portion at a time, avoiding other activities such as reading or watching television while eating.

Rewards. Asking family and friends for encouragement, setting material rewards.

Self-Monitoring. Keeping a food diary of time and place of eating, type and amount of food eaten, who was present, thought, and feelings.

Nutrition Education. Eating a healthy low-fat and high-carbohydrate diet; learning calorie values of foods.

Physical Activity. Increasing routine activity throughout the day and beginning a regular aerobic exercise program.

Cognitive Restructuring. Setting reasonable goals, thinking positive.

PHARMACOLOGICAL INTERVENTION

Some drugs decrease level of hunger or increase level of satiety. Most drugs that suppress appetite are derivatives of phenylethylamine and act on the central nervous system (Skelton, 1992). The amphetamines have potential for abuse, therefore fenfluramine HCl and phentermine HCl are preferred.

Drugs are sometimes used as adjuncts to dietary restriction. However, most licensing regulations recommend pharmacological therapy for obesity for only short periods of time, usually 12 to 16 weeks (Guy-Grand, 1992). Since weight is usually re-

gained when drug use is discontinued, short-term pharmacological therapy is ineffective.

Some investigators are now studying the effectiveness of long-term drug therapy for obesity. When other weight loss methods fail, long-term drug use may be an option. Factors to consider in selecting a drug include clinical tolerance, absence of addictive properties, sustained effects over the long-term, absence of major side effects and hazards, and known mechanism of action (Guy-Grand, 1992).

SURGERY

Surgical intervention is appropriate only for individuals with:

1. Morbid obesity (actual weight exceeding desirable weight by 100 pounds, 100 percent, or more).
2. Obesity-related medical problems.
3. A history of repeated failure with other weight loss measures (Skelton, 1992).

Before 1980, jejunoileal bypass surgery, wherein a portion of the small intestine is removed, was most commonly used. Since 1980, this type of surgery has been largely replaced by other types of surgeries because of the numerous complications and high mortality rate (Perri, 1992).

Preferred surgical interventions today are either gastroplasty (stomach stapling) or gastric bypass surgery, both of which restrict stomach size and capacity (Kral, 1992). With gastroplasty, the volume of the stomach is severely reduced to restrict the amount of food that can be eaten. A vertical line of staples in the stomach creates a 15ml pouch just beyond the gastroesophageal junction. An external band prevents expansion of the opening into the remainder of the stomach. If the patient eats too much, vomiting occurs.

One problem with gastroplasty is that some higher calorie soft foods such as cookies, chocolate, or potato chips can pass through the pouch quickly. Also, repeated overdistention can stretch the pouch. Sometimes a second surgery is necessary.

With gastric bypass surgery, the size of the stomach is reduced but the pouch is attached to a loop of the small intestine. There is greater satiety and reduced stomach capacity but gastric bypass creates malabsorption. If the patient eats too much at one time, dumping of nutrients directly from the stomach into the upper intestine can produce light-headedness, sweating, and palpitations.

Currently, gastroplasty is more common that gastric bypass surgery, but gastric bypass surgery may be slightly more effective. Surgical treatment of morbid obesity may have better long-term results than other types of treatments (Kral, 1992). However, for greatest benefit, surgical intervention must be combined with aggressive education on optimal diet and exercise habits.

EXERCISE

Regular exercise should be a part of any weight control program. Ample evidence indicates that increasing exercise increases weight loss in obese persons, especially when used in conjunction with dietary restriction (Bray, 1990; Fox, 1992). Weight loss from exercise alone rarely exceeds four to five pounds a month, but over the long-term, such losses can be significant.

For weight control, the regularity of exercise appears to be more important than the intensity, perhaps because of effects on appetite or metabolic rate (Willard, 1991). In addition, regular exercise helps preserve lean body mass with weight loss. This means that a greater portion of the weight loss is from fat as opposed to muscle. Low-intensity exercise appears to be just as effective as high-intensity exercise in preserving lean body mass (Ballor, 1990).

Regular exercise is also one of the key ingredients in weight maintenance. According to a study by Van Dale and colleagues (1990), almost all subjects who maintained a regular exercise program were moderately successful in sustaining weight loss after two years. Over 70 percent of those who did not exercise regained 75 percent or more of their weight loss.

Besides its effects on body weight, inactivity is also an independent risk factor for coronary heart disease. Exercise, with or without weight loss and dietary change, reduces risk for coronary heart disease (Fox, 1992). Exercise also improves lipid profiles, blood pressure, glucose tolerance, and enhances overall well-being.

COMMERCIAL AND POPULAR DIETS

The two main considerations in evaluating commercial and popular diets are (1) effectiveness and (2) safety. Most commercial weight loss programs are conservative in nature. However, 50 percent of those who enter commercial weight loss programs drop out within the first six weeks. At 12 weeks, drop-out rate is almost 70 percent (Perri, 1992). Of those who remain in commercial programs for longer periods, weight loss is often modest and frequently regained. The effectiveness of popular diets is usually difficult to evaluate because of their short-lived nature.

Nurses should counsel patients to avoid commercial and popular diets that do not include professional supervision, adjunct exercise or behavior modification, or a maintenance phase. Fad diets that severely restrict intake of certain foods or nutrients should also be avoided. Diets that restrict carbohydrates, salt, or fluids cause quick weight loss in a few weeks, but the loss is mostly from fluid and will quickly be regained when the patient resumes normal eating.

Dwyer (1992) recently reviewed popular diets and grouped them into three categories—reasonable, questionable, and unreasonable—according to safety of the calorie level, nutrient composition of the diet, completeness of components of the program other than diet, and cost. The results of Dwyer's review are listed in Table 5.1.

CONTRAINDICATIONS TO WEIGHT LOSS

Women who are pregnant or breast feeding should not attempt to lose weight. Likewise, children who are overweight should not be put on weight loss diets. Rather, healthy eating and exercise behaviors should be encouraged to slow the rate of weight gain and to allow height to catch up with weight.

Anorexia nervosa, bulimia, and compulsive eating disorders must be treated with psychological therapy. Successful long-term management of these conditions requires resolution of the factors driving the compulsion (Willard, 1991).

The next chapter will provide a primer on good nutrition. The latest food guides and dietary guidelines will be discussed to set the context for developing individualized diet plans.

Table 5.1 Some Reasonable, Questionable, and Unreasonable Diets for the Treatment of Obesity

1200 calories per day or more
Reasonable diets

I Don't Eat (But I Can't Lose) Weight Control Program
Harvard Square Diet
Red Book Wise Women's Diet
Doctor's Calorie Plus
Behavior Control Diet
California Nutrition Book
California Diet
LEARN Program for Weight Control
Complete University Medical Diet

Questionable diets

Oat and Wheat Bran Health Plan
New Canadian Fiber Diet (DePrey)
Women's Advantage Diet (Mallek)
The 35 Plus Diet for Women
Bad Back Diet Book (Green and Ceresa)
"T" Factor Diet
The Mediterranean Diet
Atkin's Diet Revolution
Nutrition Breakthrough
Dr. Abravanel's Body Type Diet
Doctor's Quick Weight Loss
Pritikin Program Diet
Craig Claibourne's Gourmet Diet
Rechtschaffen Diet
Orthocarbohydrate Diet
Easy No Risk Diet
Slender Now
Never Say Diet
F Plan Diet
Carbohydrate Craver's Diet
Dr. Atkin's Health Revolution
Immune Power
What Your Doctor Didn't Learn in Medical School

800 to 1199 calories per day
Reasonable diets

Lean and Green Diet
Hilton Head Metabolism Diet
Weight Watcher's Quick Start Program
Diet Workshop Lo Carbo and Beacon Hill Diets

Questionable diets

Two Day Diet
Rotation Diet
Diet Workshop Wild Weekend
The Hilton Head Over 35 Diet
L. A. Diet
Doctor's Metabolic Diet
No Choice Diet
Woman Doctor's Diet
Southhampton Diet
Bloomingdale Diet
Herbalife Slim Trim Diet
Fit for Life
Thin So Fast (Eades)
The Rice Diet
Beverly Hills Diet

800 calories or less
Reasonable diets (only if administered under medical supervision)

HMR (Health Management Resources)
Optifast
United Weight Control
New Directions (Ross Laboratories)
Nutrisystem

Questionable diets

Herbalife
Last Chance Diet
Fasting Is A Way of Life

Source: Dwyer, J.T. (1992). "Treatment of obesity: Conventional programs and fad diets." In P. Bjorntorp and B.N. Brodoff (Eds.), *Obesity* (pp.662–676). Philadelphia: J.B. Lippincott Co. Reprinted with permission.

EXAM QUESTIONS

Chapter 5

Questions 40-48

40. What percentage of obese individuals have mild obesity:

    a. 60%
    b. 70%
    c. 80%
    d. 90%

41. Mild obesity is best treated with?

    a. a balanced, low-caloric diet
    b. a very low-caloric diet
    c. exercise only
    d. behavior modification only

42. Weight loss is achieved when:

    a. the balance of calories taken in and calories expended does not affect weight loss
    b. calories taken in are greater than calories expended
    c. calories taken in are balanced with calories expended
    d. calories taken in are fewer than calories expended

43. Which of the following is not an important element of behavior modification?

    a. stimulus control
    b. self-monitoring
    c. cognitive restructuring
    d. psychotherapy

44. For which of the following groups is weight loss contraindicated?

    a. children
    b. young adults
    c. older adults
    d. weight loss is not contraindicated for any group

45. Very low-calorie diets may be appropriate for patients who exceed desirable body weight by what percentage?

    a. 20% or more
    b. 100% or more
    c. 60% or more
    d. 40% or more

46. Surgery may be appropriate for patients who exceed desirable body weight by what percentage?

    a. 150% or more
    b. 60% or more
    c. 40% or more
    d. 100% or more

47. An appropriate weight loss goal for obese individuals would be to lose:

    a. 5% of current body weight for any single treatment course
    b. 10-15% of current body weight for any single treatment course
    c. 25% of current body weight for any single treatment course
    d. entire percentage of desirable body weight according to weight for height tables

48. Balanced, low-calorie diets usually provide what level of calorie intake daily?

    a. about 2,000 calories
    b. 600 to 800 calories
    c. less than 1,000 calories
    d. 1,000 to 1,500 calories

CHAPTER 6

DIET INTERVENTION
A NUTRITION PRIMER

CHAPTER OBJECTIVE

After reading this chapter, you will be able to recognize the nutritional components of a balanced diet and describe how macronutrients and micronutrients help maintain overall good health.

LEARNING OBJECTIVES

After studying this chapter you will able to:

1. Specify common nutrient excesses and deficiencies in the American diet.

2. Describe the latest nutritional recommendations, dietary guidelines, and food guides.

INTRODUCTION

An understanding of basic nutrition concepts will help nurses to assist with nutritional counseling of patients and to design diet plans. This chapter will explain the role of protein, carbohydrate, fat, vitamins, minerals, and water in a balanced diet. The Recommended Dietary Allowances and food sources for nutrients will be given. The chapter will also explain how to translate these recommendations into food choices for good health using both the Dietary Guidelines for Americans and the New Food Guide Pyramid.

OVERVIEW

Good nutrition means providing the body with the right balance of nutrients for optimal functioning. The human body has an amazing capacity to synthesize hundreds of chemical compounds for use. Forty or so of these compounds, or nutrients, serve as raw materials or catalysts for metabolic processes, and must be supplied by food.

The major nutrient categories include carbohydrates, fats, protein, minerals, vitamins, and water. Nutrients are released from food through the digestive system and absorbed. Some are chemically altered, and all are transported via the blood to the body cells.

There are two main types of nutrients (1) *macronutrients* and (2) *micronutrients*. The macronutrients are protein, carbohydrate, and fat. Among other functions, these nutrients provide the body with calories that can be burned for fuel. Although not essential, alcohol also provides calories. The micronutrients include vitamins and minerals. Vitamins and minerals do not provide calories but are essential for life, as is water.

Of the macronutrients, fat is the most concentrated source of calories. Fat provides nine calories per gram as compared to four calories per gram for carbohydrate or protein. Alcohol is also a fairly concentrated source of calories at seven calories per gram. All three macronutrients—carbohydrates, proteins, and fats can be metabolized to release energy. In most diets, carbohydrates and fats are the primary sources of energy, which allows the body to use protein for synthesis and maintenance of body systems. When carbohydrates and fats aren't available for energy from food, the body turns to its stores of fat, dietary protein, and finally uses its own tissue to meet energy needs.

In our affluent society, finding a nutritious diet might not seem to be a problem. But for most Americans, the major problem isn't the scarcity of food or severe lack of specific types of foods or even ingredients. The problem is the overconsumption of food, leading to excess storage of fat and resultant obesity.

Although Americans have access to healthful and nutritious foods, choices of food are often poor. Americans tend to eat too much fat, saturated fat, cholesterol, protein, and refined sugars, and too little carbohydrate and fiber. In her book, *The Complete University Medical Diet*, Dr. Simonson (1983) notes the following:

> The average American eats 55 tons of food by the time he is 70. This amounts to 29 tons of solid food, washed down by 6,500 gallons of liquid (of which 2,200 is coffee). It includes 9 pigs, 8 cows, and 15,000 eggs.

PROTEIN

Proteins make up the major structural components of animal cells, and are nicknamed "the building blocks of life." Protein is the only substance that is capable of building and repairing cells and tissues. It is the major building material for muscles, blood, skin, nails, and internal organs, including the heart and brain.

All forms of life, from microscopic forms to man, have their own characteristic proteins. Yet, all proteins are formed from the same 20 or so relatively simple amino acids. Amino acids are strung together like links on a chain and then wound into various shapes. Each animal species forms characteristic proteins, and within a species the protein of each animal is unique.

Proteins in the form of enzymes are needed to catalyze and control all metabolic reactions. Proteins perform the following metabolic functions: they provide raw materials for synthesis of antibodies and some hormones; they regulate fluid balance; they transport fats; they provide heat and energy; they regulate acid-base balance; and they provide raw material for synthesis of enzymes, to build and repair tissue.

The body is able to convert some amino acids into other amino acids. There are eight essential amino acids that can only come from the diet. Animal proteins are composed of amino acids that are similar to human proteins, and form a good source of essential amino acids. Plant proteins do not contain all the essential amino acids but can be combined for complete protein.

Most Americans eat more than the recommended daily allowances of protein. In sedentary people, excessive consumption of animal protein with high fat content can lead to obesity and other health problems (Bray, 1985).

Animal proteins in meat, poultry, fish, eggs, milk, and cheese contain all the essential amino acids and are considered high-quality proteins. Plant proteins do not contain all the essential amino acids, but can be combined with other plant proteins to provide complete protein.

In general, combining foods in two of the following three plant food groups—dried beans and peas, grain products, or nuts and seeds—will yield a complete protein. Examples of such combinations include a peanut butter and jelly sandwich or a dish of beans and rice. Combining a small amount of animal protein with a plant protein will also complete the plant protein. An example of this combination would be a cheese sandwich or split pea soup with ham.

In a balanced diet, protein should provide 12 to 20 percent of calories. However, many Americans eat almost twice as much protein as they need. In sedentary individuals, excessive consumption of animal foods that are high in protein but also high in fat (such as fatty cuts of red meat, fried meats, whole milk, and high-fat cheeses) can lead to obesity and other health problems (Bray, 1985).

CARBOHYDRATE

Contrary to popular belief, carbohydrates are not fattening. Carbohydrates contain less than one-half the calories of fat per equal weight unit. There are two main types of carbohydrates—*simple* and *complex*. Simple carbohydrates include naturally occurring sugars found in fruits, vegetables, and milk, and refined sugars such as sucrose. Complex carbohydrates include starch and dietary fiber. Dietary fiber promotes laxation and improves several metabolic

functions in the body, but is not fully digested and thus provides minimal calories.

Carbohydrates are the body's main fuel source. The brain relies on glucose to provide it with fuel. Carbohydrates help in body functions, such as digestion, and muscle exertion, while helping us function and think clearly.

Carbohydrates produce the energy needed for body work, and in most cultures, carbohydrates supply most of the energy requirements of humans. Some carbohydrates are required to form a structural component of certain body compounds while others help regulate normal metabolic functions.

Starches from grains and root vegetables have traditionally been man's main source of carbohydrates. Starches and sugars are broken down during digestion into small soluble molecules that can be absorbed from the bloodstream and transported to the cells. Glucose, a simple chemical substance, is the main product of these digestive processes. Chemical reactions within the cells release the energy in the glucose molecule so that it can be used for work and heat.

Sugar, as sucrose, is a relatively new addition to the diet. High sucrose levels in the body have been linked with many health problems, including dental caries and atherosclerosis. The lure of sugar has also been linked to overeating and increased fat storage leading to obesity. Carbohydrates are digested more quickly than other nutrients.

Carbohydrates generally make up about 45 to 50 percent of calories in a typical American diet. However, recommended levels of carbohydrate intake are 55 to 60 percent of calories. Therefore, Americans need to eat more carbohydrate-rich foods such as fruits, vegetables, grain products, dried beans, and peas.

FAT

Although "fat" may conjure up a negative image, fats, or lipids, are essential to any diet. They form the most concentrated form of energy available to the body. Fats are made up of long chains of chemical compounds termed fatty acids, which are chemically bonded to a molecule of the alcohol glycerol. During digestion, these complex fats are broken down into simpler substances that can be absorbed through the digestive tract, transported to cells, and then used for energy or recombined into fat for storage in the cells.

Some stored fat is essential for good health. It provides a ready energy source during stress, helps insulate the body from environmental changes, and acts as a cushion around vital organs, protecting them from physical shock. Fats keep the skin soft and supple, contribute to healthy hair, act as a reserve source of fuel, as a lubricant, and also help the body break down and utilize fat-soluble vitamins.

Fat has the following metabolic functions. It provides heat and energy, protects and insulates, and is a structural component of all cells. Fat provides raw materials for synthesis of some vital compounds, and acts as an energy-storage depot as well.

Whereas fat is necessary for health maintenance, most Americans eat too much fat. The typical American diet contains about 40 percent of calories or more as fat (Connor, 1986). The recommended amount is no more than 30 percent of calories as fat. Fortunately, the foods high in complex carbohydrates and naturally occurring sugars that Americans need to eat more of are also low in fat.

Plant and animal foods contain fat. There are three main types of fats in the diet—*saturated fats, monounsaturated fats,* and *polyunsaturated fats.* Saturated fats are solid at room temperature. At the molecular level they contain no double bonds between carbon atoms. Animal fats generally are saturated. Palm and coconut oil are also saturated. Saturated fats raise blood cholesterol levels and clog arteries.

Monounsaturated fats contain one double bond between carbon atoms. Monounsaturated fats are liquid at room temperature and may help lower blood cholesterol levels. Olive oil and canola oil are good sources of monounsaturated fats.

Polyunsaturated fats contain multiple double bonds between carbon atoms and are also liquid at room temperature. Most plant oils such as corn, safflower, soybean, and sunflower oil are polyunsaturated. However, solid margarines and shortenings made from plant oils are partially hydrogenated, that is, hydrogen atoms are added to the molecule at the site of the double bonds, making these fats more like saturated fats. Thus liquid or tub margarines are preferable to stick margarines.

Another type of polyunsaturated fat, omega-3 fatty acids, are found in fish oils. The omega-3 fats are one of the few unsaturated fats of animal origin. Many studies show that omega-3 fatty acids lower blood triglyceride levels dramatically and blood cholesterol levels modestly. They may also lower risk of heart disease by prolonging clotting time. Fatty fish like salmon, mackerel, haddock, trout, and herring are rich in omega-3 fatty acids.

Although monounsaturated fats and polyunsaturated fats do not raise blood cholesterol levels as saturated fats do, they are still fats and a very concentrated source of calories. Americans need to reduce intake of total fat as well as saturated fat.

Cholesterol is a fatlike substance that is essential for many body functions. However, it is not a nutrient because our bodies can make cholesterol. But when we eat too much cholesterol and saturated fat, our bodies make even more cholesterol, raising blood cholesterol levels and increasing risk for heart disease.

Cholesterol is found only in animal foods; plant foods contain no cholesterol. Eggs yolks and organ meats are particularly concentrated sources of cholesterol. Fattier cuts of red meat and high-fat dairy products are also high in cholesterol. Shellfish such as shrimp, crab, and lobster are not as high in cholesterol as previously thought.

ALCOHOL

Alcohol provides seven calories per gram, so it is a fairly concentrated source of calories. Alcoholic beverages provide almost no vitamins or minerals and many calories, so they are poor choices for individuals trying to lose weight. Alcoholic beverages often replace other more nutritious foods, leading to poor nutritional content of the diet. In addition, alcohol can raise blood triglyceride levels, which may be a risk factor for heart disease for some people.

Some studies in the past have suggested that drinking a small amount of alcohol each day raises high-density lipoprotein cholesterol levels, which protect against heart disease. However, recent studies have cast doubt on this theory. Women who are pregnant or trying to conceive should avoid alcohol entirely, since even modest alcohol use during pregnancy can cause birth defects.

VITAMINS

Few groups of nutrients have caught the researcher's attention with such fervor as vitamins, particularly vitamins C and E.

Vitamins were the last nutrients discovered and have probably been the subject of more interest and controversy than any other single group of nutrients. Beginning in 1900, vitamins quickly caught the imagination of the general public. In more recent years, scientists have sought to prove that, for some vitamins, "more is better." Vitamins C and E are good cases in point.

What are vitamins? According to Williams (1976), there are two characteristics that make a compound a vitamin:

1. It must be a vital organic dietary substance, which is neither carbohydrate, fat, nor protein, and is necessary only in very small quantities to do special metabolic jobs or to prevent deficiency disease.

2. It cannot be manufactured by the body and therefore must be supplied via food.

With more data, it is now apparent that at least one compound, vitamin D, is misassigned to the vitamin group. It behaves like a hormone.

Vitamins are also usually grouped according to solubility in a medium. The fat-soluble vitamins, A, D, E, and K, are closely associated with lipids, while the water-soluble vitamins, B complex and C, are absorbed and transported more easily throughout the body. The following list contains sources of the fat- and water-soluble vitamins.

FOODS RICH IN VITAMINS

Vitamin C: Citrus fruits, cantaloupe, strawberries, broccoli, green leafy vegetables, tomatoes

B vitamins:

Thiamine (B1): Dried peas and beans, meats (especially pork), cereals (whole-grain or enriched), nuts

Riboflavin (B2): Liver, milk, cheese, eggs, green leafy vegetables

Niacin: Liver, meats, dried peas and beans, cereals (whole-grain or enriched)

Pyridoxine (B6): Liver, meats, wheat germ, whole-grain cereals

Folic acid: Liver, yeast, green leafy vegetables, dried peas and beans, nuts, whole-grain cereals

Cobalamin (B12): Liver and other organ meats, meats, eggs, milk, and milk products

Vitamin A: Liver, butter, eggs, whole milk, green and yellow vegetables

Vitamin D: Fish liver oils, milk fortified with vitamin D, sunlight

Vitamin E: Wheat germ, whole grains, vegetable oils, eggs, whole milk, liver

Vitamin K: Green leafy vegetables, egg yolk, soybean oil, liver

Source: Stuart and Davis, *Slim Chance in a Fat World*, 1972.

Disease caused by vitamin deficiency is rare in the United States. Although many Americans take vitamin and minerals supplements, there is no evidence that taking more than the required amount of vitamin or mineral will improve health. Taking too much of certain vitamins or minerals can be harmful. If use of a vitamin or mineral supplement is indicated, patients should be counseled to select one with a broad base of vitamins and minerals provided at low doses supplying approximately 100 percent of the Recommended Dietary Allowances.

MINERALS

Unlike vitamins, which are compounds, minerals occur singly as elements. Only about 4 percent of the body is composed of minerals, yet these nutrients have very important metabolic roles. The structural function of calcium, phosphorus, and small amounts of other elements is readily seen in the bones and teeth. Minerals are essential for some enzyme actions, the regulation of fluid balance, nerve transmissions, muscle contractions, acid-base balance, and as a component of some vital compounds.

Minerals are important components of some body compounds, such as the iron in hemoglobin and iodine in thyroxine. Many enzymes have mineral elements, such as copper, zinc, and molybdenum, incorporated into molecular structures. They may require the presence of such minerals as magnesium to complete chemical reactions.

Macrominerals are those minerals needed in amounts above 100mg per day. Microminerals, or trace elements, are needed in smaller amounts.

These are macrominerals: calcium, chloride, magnesium, phosphorus, potassium, sodium, and sulfur. The microminerals are arsenic, cadmium (possibly), chromium, cobalt, copper, fluoride, iodine, iron, manganese, molybdenum, nickel, selenium, silicon, tin, vanadium, and zinc.

For certain groups of Americans, intake of calcium, iron, magnesium, and zinc is somewhat less than the recommended levels. Rich food sources of some of the minerals are listed below:

Calcium: Milk, cheese, sardines, ice cream, green leafy vegetables (except for spinach, beet greens, and chard)

Phosphorus: Liver, milk, meat, cheese, cereals, eggs

Iodine: Seafood, vegetables (grown in soil with adequate iodine levels), iodized salt

Iron: Liver, meat, dried fruits, green leafy vegetables

Magnesium: Green leafy vegetables, nuts, whole-grain cereals, dried peas and beans

Potassium: Bananas, oranges, tomatoes, potatoes, broccoli, and some meats

Zinc: Eggs, oysters, liver, meats, poultry, legumes, and nuts

Chromium: Brewer's yeast, grain and cereal products

FIBER

Fiber is the part of plant foods that is not fully digested in the body. Only plant foods contain fiber; animal foods contain no fiber. There are two main types of fiber, *soluble* and *insoluble* fiber. Both types of fiber are important for good health.

Insoluble fiber is found in unrefined wheat and most other types of whole cereal grains. Soluble fiber is found in dried beans and peas and oat products. Fruits and vegetables contain both soluble and insoluble fiber. Insoluble fiber aids bowel regularity. Soluble fiber lowers blood fat levels and stabilizes blood sugar.

WATER

Water, the most plentiful compound in the body, is too often overlooked. The body is composed of 50 to 75 percent water. This remarkable fluid is not only the major ingredient in blood, but is also actively involved in nearly every body function. Water carries and supplies nutrients, participates in chemical reactions, disposes of waste products, and regulates the body's temperature as it continually bathes the cells (Ferguson, 1983). While men and women have existed for weeks without food, most people can't survive longer than about 10 days without water. When water intake is inadequate, the organs and glands cannot function properly, and the body's wastes aren't washed out of the system.

Water forms one of the basic ingredients in many diet programs. Each day, the body loses large amounts of water through breathing, perspiration, urination, and other body processes. Under most circumstances, the body will continue to excrete these amounts no matter what water intake is.

Most dietary programs recommend drinking eight 8oz. glasses of water per day. Increasing this amount in very hot weather or during strenuous exercise is recommended.

THE RECOMMENDED DIETARY ALLOWANCES

As Stuart and Davis (1972) have noted, each cell is surrounded by a nutrient sea, and it selects just what it needs to perform its own specific task. While it's impossible to determine exact cellular needs, scientists can only estimate the amount of nutrients needed to prevent clinical signs of nutritional deficiencies. Suggested amounts are based on these estimates, plus an added "safety allowance," or a margin of nutritional safety. In the United States the National Research Council of the National Academy of Sciences has developed a table of suggested dietary allowances, or the Recommended Dietary Allowances (RDA). These tables are updated and revised as more knowledge is gained. The RDAs consider the fact that individuals vary widely in their nutritional requirements. The recommendations are thus intended to cover the needs not only of the average person but of most healthy persons.

The RDA's are defined as "the level of intake of essential nutrients that, on the basis of scientific knowledge, are judged by the Food and Nutrition Board to be adequate to meet the known nutrient needs of practically all healthy persons (Food and Nutrition Board of the National Research Council, 1989)."

As shown in Table 6.1, the RDA varies according to age groups, with separate categories for pregnant and lactating women. In addition to the RDA, the Food and Nutrition Board also establishes estimated safe and adequate daily intake of certain vitamins and minerals (Table 6.2). The board makes such estimations when enough data are available to set safe ranges but not absolute requirements. The RDA can serve as a standard for evaluating the nutritional adequacy of diets.

DIETARY GUIDELINES FOR AMERICANS

The U.S. Departments of Agriculture and Health and Human Services (1990) give seven guidelines to foster healthy eating for Americans. Guidelines similar to these were first published in the late 1970s and have been updated as more is learned about nutrition and disease. The seven guidelines are:

1. *Eat a variety of foods.* No single type of food supplies all essential nutrients in the amounts needed. Variety in the diet is so important that it should be repeatedly emphasized. Variety helps maximize the chances that all the essential nutrients will be included in the diet, and also minimizes the chance that any one mineral or nutrient will be used in overly large proportions.

2. *Maintain ideal weight.* Being overweight increases the chance of developing chronic conditions such as high blood pressure, heart disease, stroke, type II diabetes, certain cancers, and other illnesses. Gradual weight loss through a balanced low-calorie diet and exercise is recommended.

3. *Choose a diet low in fat, saturated fat, and cholesterol.* Diets that are high in fat, saturated fat, and cholesterol increase blood cholesterol levels. Moderate intake of fat and cholesterol is a sensible approach. People don't have to eliminate certain foods from their diet, rather, they should eat high-fat and high-cholesterol foods in moderation.

Here are some hints to reduce fat and cholesterol intake:

Fats and oils:
- Use fats and oils sparingly in cooking.
- Use small amounts of salad dressings and spreads.

Table 6.1 Recommended Dietary Allowances[a]

Category	Age (years) or Condition	Weight[b] (kg)	(lb)	Height[b] (cm)	(in)	Protein (g)	Fat-Soluble Vitamins — Vita-min A (μg RE)[c]	Vita-min D (μg)[d]	Vita-min E (mg α-TE)[e]	Vita-min K (μg)	Water-Soluble Vitamins — Vita-min C (mg)	Thia-min (mg)	Ribo-flavin (mg)	Niacin (mg NE)[f]	Vita-min B6 (mg)	Fo-late (μg)	Vitamin B12 (μg)	Minerals — Cal-cium (mg)	Phos-phorus (mg)	Mag-nesium (mg)	Iron (mg)	Zinc (mg)	Iodine (μg)	Sele-nium (μg)
Infants	0.0–0.5	6	13	60	24	13	375	7.5	3	5	30	0.3	0.4	5	0.3	25	0.3	400	300	40	6	5	40	10
	0.5–1.0	9	20	71	28	14	375	10	4	10	35	0.4	0.5	6	0.6	35	0.5	600	500	60	10	5	50	15
Children	1–3	13	29	90	35	16	400	10	6	15	40	0.7	0.8	9	1.0	50	0.7	800	800	80	10	10	70	20
	4–6	20	44	112	44	24	500	10	7	20	45	0.9	1.1	12	1.1	75	1.0	800	800	120	10	10	90	20
	7–10	28	62	132	52	28	700	10	7	30	45	1.0	1.2	13	1.4	100	1.4	800	800	170	10	10	120	30
Males	11–14	45	99	157	62	45	1,000	10	10	45	50	1.3	1.5	17	1.7	150	2.0	1,200	1,200	270	12	15	150	40
	15–18	66	145	176	69	59	1,000	10	10	65	60	1.5	1.8	20	2.0	200	2.0	1,200	1,200	400	12	15	150	50
	19–24	72	160	177	70	58	1,000	10	10	70	60	1.5	1.7	19	2.0	200	2.0	1,200	1,200	350	10	15	150	70
	25–50	79	174	176	70	63	1,000	5	10	80	60	1.5	1.7	19	2.0	200	2.0	800	800	350	10	15	150	70
	51+	77	170	173	68	63	1,000	5	10	80	60	1.2	1.4	15	2.0	200	2.0	800	800	350	10	15	150	70
Females	11–14	46	101	157	62	46	800	10	8	45	50	1.1	1.3	15	1.4	150	2.0	1,200	1,200	280	15	12	150	45
	15–18	55	120	163	64	44	800	10	8	55	60	1.1	1.3	15	1.5	180	2.0	1,200	1,200	300	15	12	150	50
	19–24	58	128	164	65	46	800	10	8	60	60	1.1	1.3	15	1.6	180	2.0	1,200	1,200	280	15	12	150	55
	25–50	63	138	163	64	50	800	5	8	65	60	1.1	1.3	15	1.6	180	2.0	800	800	280	15	12	150	55
	51+	65	143	160	63	50	800	5	8	65	60	1.0	1.2	13	1.6	180	2.0	800	800	280	10	12	150	55
Pregnant						60	800	10	10	65	70	1.5	1.6	17	2.2	400	2.2	1,200	1,200	320	30	15	175	65
Lactating	1st 6 months					65	1,300	10	12	65	95	1.6	1.8	20	2.1	280	2.6	1,200	1,200	355	15	19	200	75
	2nd 6 months					62	1,200	10	11	65	90	1.6	1.7	20	2.1	260	2.6	1,200	1,200	340	15	16	200	75

[a] The allowances, expressed as average daily intakes over time, are intended to provide for individual variations among most normal persons as they live in the United States under usual environmental stresses. Diets should be based on a variety of common foods in order to provide other nutrients for which human requirements have been less well defined. See text for detailed discussion of allowances and of nutrients not tabulated.

[b] Weights and heights of Reference Adults are actual medians for the U.S. population of the designated age, as reported by NHANES II. The median weights and heights of those under 19 years of age were taken from Hamill et al. (1979) (see pages 16–17). The use of these figures does not imply that the height-to-weight ratios are ideal.

[c] Retinol equivalents. 1 retinol equivalent = 1 μg retinol or 6 μg β-carotene. See text for calculation of vitamin A activity of diets as retinol equivalents.

[d] As cholecalciferol. 10 μg cholecalciferol = 400 IU of vitamin D.

[e] α-Tocopherol equivalents. 1 mg d-α tocopherol = 1 α-TE. See text for variation in allowances and calculation of vitamin E activity of the diet as α-tocopherol equivalents.

[f] 1 NE (niacin equivalent) is equal to 1 mg of niacin or 60 mg of dietary tryptophan.

Source: Food and Nutrition Board, National Research Council. Reprinted with permission from *Recommended Dietary Allowances, 10th Edition.* Copyright 1989 by the National Academy of Sciences. Courtesy of the National Academy Press, Washington, D.C.

Table 6.2 SUMMARY TABLE. Estimated Safe and Adequate Daily Dietary Intakes of Selected Vitamins and Minerals[a]

Category	Age (Years)	Vitamins Biotin (µg)	Panthothenic Acid (mg)
Infants	0–0.5	10	2
	0.5–1	15	3
Children and adolescents	1–3	20	3
	4–6	25	3–4
	7–10	30	4–5
	11+	30–100	4–7
Adults		30–100	4–7

Category	Age (years)	Trace Elements[b] Copper (mg)	Manganese (mg)	Flouride (mg)	Chromium (µg)	Molybdenum (µg)
Infants	0–0.5	0.4–0.6	0.3–0.6	0.1–0.5	10–10	15–30
	0.5–1	0.6–0.7	0.6–1.0	0.2–1.0	20–60	20–40
Children and adolescents	1–3	0.7–1.0	1.0–1.5	0.5–1.5	20–80	25–50
	4–6	1.0–1.5	1.5–2.0	1.0–2.5	30–120	30–75
	7–10	1.0–2.0	2.0–3.0	1.5–2.5	50–200	50–150
	11+	1.5–2.5	2.0–5.0	1.5–2.5	50–200	75–250
Adults		1.5–3.0	2.0–5.0	1.5–4.0	50–200	75–250

[a]Because there is less information on which to base allowances, these figures are not given in the main table of RDA and are provided here in the form of ranges of recommended intakes.

[b] Since the toxic levels for many trace elements may be only several times usual intakes, the upper levels for the trace elements given in this table should not be habitually exceeded.

Source: Food and Nutrition Board, National Research Council. Reprinted with permission from *Recommended Dietary Allowances, 10th Edition*. Copyright 1989 by the National Academy of Sciences. Courtesy of the National Academy Press, Washington, D.C.

- Choose liquid vegetables oils.
- Read labels to learn food content.

Meat, poultry, fish, dry beans, and eggs:
- Eat two to three servings, or about six ounces daily.
- Trim fat from meat and remove skin from poultry.
- Use dried beans and peas in place of meat.
- Moderate the use of eggs yolks and organ meats.

Milk and milk products:
- Eat two to three servings daily (one serving equals 1 cup of milk or yogurt or 1 1/2 ounce cheese).
- Choose skim, low-fat, or fat-free products.

4. *Choose a diet with plenty of vegetables, fruits, and grain products.* Adults should eat at least three servings of vegetables and two servings of fruits daily. Adults should eat at least six servings daily of grain products such as breads, cereals, pasta, and rice. Whenever possible, choose whole grain products to increase fiber intake. Dried beans and peas are also rich in carbohydrate and fiber and low in fat.

5. *Use sugars only in moderation.* Simple carbohydrates, such as sugars and products made with large amounts of sugar and syrups, provide little more than excess calories. Sugars promote tooth decay and aren't really needed in the diet.

To avoid excess sugar in the diet, try

- Using less of all types of sugars, including white sugar, brown sugar, raw sugar, honey, and syrups.

- Using fewer foods containing these types of sugars, including candies, soft drinks, ice cream, cakes, and cookies.

- Selecting fresh fruits, fruits canned without sugar, or fruits canned in light syrup rather than in heavy syrup. Many canned fruits are now preserved in their own juice; remember, however, that the allowance for fresh fruits is twice that for canned fruits.

- Read labels for information about sugar content in particular foods. Look for terms such as sucrose, glucose, maltose, dextrose, lactose, fructose, or syrups, all of which are largely sugar.

6. *Use salt and sodium only in moderation.* Most Americans eat too much salt. Excessive sodium in the diet can be associated with increased risk of developing hypertension. Reducing the amount of sodium in the diet may also help lower elevated blood pressure.

Most types of food, except fruits in their natural state, provide some sodium. Table salt, preservatives, leavening agents, and certain flavoring agents markedly increase the amount of sodium in the diet. In addition, many of the over-the-counter drugs contain significant amounts of sodium and need to be considered as well. The best measure is to read all labels carefully.

Ways to cut down the amount of sodium in the diet include

- Cook with only small amounts of salt or no salt.

- Use spices and herbs instead of salt (see Chapter 10).
- Add little or no salt to food at the table.

- Limit the use of overly salty foods, which include some of everyone's favorites—potato chips, pretzels, nuts, and popcorn, condiments such as soy sauce, steak sauce, garlic salt, processed cheese, and luncheon meats.

Some people have special health problems that demand a slightly different approach to dieting and use of certain foods. In the next chapter, we'll look at the special nutritional needs of persons with diabetes, those at risk of cardiovascular disease, and hypertension. In addition, we'll discuss some of the special considerations that must be made when designing a diet for an elderly overweight patient.

7. *If you drink alcoholic beverages, do so in moderation.* Alcoholic beverages contain calories but are virtually void of nutrients. If adults decide to drink alcoholic beverages, no more than one drink a day is recommended for women and no more than two a day for men. One drink is considered 12 ounces of beer, five ounces of wine, or 1 1/2 ounces of distilled spirits (80 proof).

Some people should not drink alcoholic beverages at all. These include:

- Women who are pregnant or trying to conceive.
- Individuals who are planning to drive or do another activity that requires skill and concentration.
- Individuals taking certain medicines.
- Individuals who cannot control their drinking.
- Children and adolescents.

THE NEW FOOD GUIDE PYRAMID

The U.S. Department of Agriculture (1992) recently introduced a new food guide to replace the basic four food groups and serve as a guide for implementing the Dietary Guidelines for Americans. As shown in Figure 6.1, the pyramid recommends ample servings of grains, fruits, and vegetables and more limited servings of dairy products, protein foods, and fats.

Some patients may be surprised by the quantities of food suggested by this guide. When less fat is eaten, they discover that they can eat a much greater volume of food. Women and some older adults should eat the smaller number of servings of the ranges given in the pyramid, while very active individuals and teenagers can eat more servings. For controlling calories, choose lower-calorie foods in each group and limit the top group, fats, sweets and oils. Table 6.3 shows what counts as a serving for each food group.

The next chapter will give some guidelines for designing specific diets for individuals trying to lose weight.

Table 6.3 What counts as one serving?

Breads, Cereal, Rice, and Pasta

1 slice of bread
1/2 cup of cooked rice or pasta
1/2 cup of cooked cereal
1 ounce of ready-to-eat cereal

Vegetables

1/2 cup of chopped raw or cooked vegetables
1 cup of leafy raw vegetables

Fruits

1 piece of fruit or melon wedge
3/4 cup of juice
1/2 cup of canned fruit
1/4 cup of dried fruit

Milk, Yogurt, and Cheese

1 cup of milk or yogurt
1–1/2 to 2 ounces of cheese

Meat, Poultry, Fish, Dry Beans, Eggs, and Nuts

2–1/2 to 3 ounces of cooked lean meat, poultry, or fish
Count 1/2 cup of cooked beans, or 1 egg, or 2 tablespoons of peanut butter as 1 ounce of lean meat (about 1/3 serving)

Source: U.S. Department of Agriculture, Human Nutrition Information Service, August 1992, Leaflet No. 572.

A Guide to Daily Food Choices

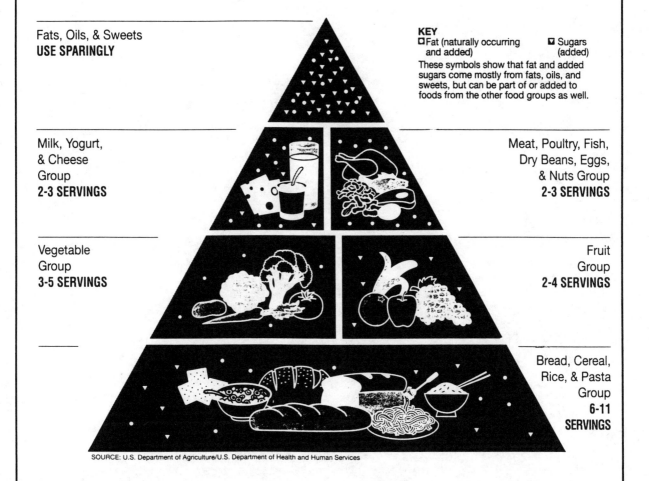

Fats, Oils, & Sweets
USE SPARINGLY

KEY
☐ Fat (naturally occurring   ◨ Sugars
  and added)   (added)
These symbols show that fat and added
sugars come mostly from fats, oils, and
sweets, but can be part of or added to
foods from the other food groups as well.

Milk, Yogurt,
& Cheese
Group
2-3 SERVINGS

Meat, Poultry, Fish,
Dry Beans, Eggs,
& Nuts Group
2-3 SERVINGS

Vegetable
Group
3-5 SERVINGS

Fruit
Group
2-4 SERVINGS

Bread, Cereal,
Rice, & Pasta
Group
**6-11
SERVINGS**

SOURCE: U.S. Department of Agriculture/U.S. Department of Health and Human Services

Use the Food Guide Pyramid to help you eat better every day. . .the Dietary Guidelines way. Start with plenty of Breads, Cereals, Rice, and Pasta; Vegetables; and Fruits. Add two to three servings from the Milk group and two to three servings from the Meat group.

Each of these food groups provides some, but not all, of the nutrients you need. No one food group is more important than another — for good health you need them all. Go easy on fats, oils, and sweets, the foods in the small tip of the Pyramid.

Figure 6.1 The Food Guide Pyramid.

Source: **U.S. Department of Agriculture, Human Nutrition Information Service, August 1992, Leaflet No. 572.**

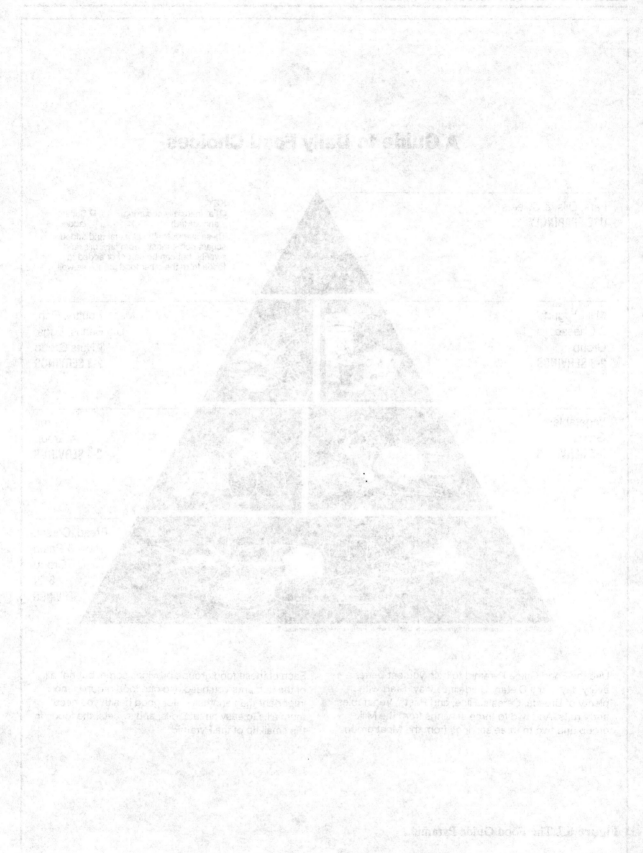

EXAM QUESTIONS

Chapter 6

Questions 49-58

49. Under the New Food Guide Pyramid, how many servings from the bread, cereal, rice, and pasta groups are recommended daily?

    a. 1
    b. 2-3
    c. 4-5
    d. 6-11

50. Fat should provide what percentage of total calorie intake in a balanced diet?

    a. 40% or less
    b. 30% or less
    c. 20% or less
    d. 10% or less

51. Protein should provide what percentage of total calorie intake in a balanced diet?

    a. 12-20%
    b. 25-28%
    c. 30-38%
    d. 50% or more

52. Protein, carbohydrate, and fat are referred to as:

    a. micronutrients
    b. macronutrients
    c. meganutrients
    d. complex nutrients

53. Which of the following contains the most energy per gram?

    a. protein
    b. alcohol
    c. carbohydrate
    d. fat

54. Calcium is considered a:

    a. macronutrient
    b. macromineral
    c. micromineral
    d. vitamin

55. Which type of fat tends to raise blood cholesterol levels?

    a. saturated fat
    b. monounsaturated fat
    c. polyunsaturated fat
    d. omega-3 fatty acids

56. Which of the following should be the major energy source in a balanced diet?

    a. vitamins and minerals
    b. carbohydrate
    c. fat
    d. protein

57. Which of the following is a good source of vitamin C?

    a. broccoli
    b. liver
    c. yeast
    d. fish oil

58. The level of intake of essential nutrients judged o meet the needs of most healthy individuals is called:

    a. Recommended Dietary Allowances
    b. Minimum Daily Requirements
    c. Basal Metabolic Requirements
    d. Nutrient Index

CHAPTER 7

DIET INTERVENTION DESIGNING DIET PLANS

CHAPTER OBJECTIVE

After studying this chapter, you will be able identify characteristics of a balanced, low-calorie diet and select an appropriate calorie level and nutrient composition.

LEARNING OBJECTIVES

After studying this chapter, you will be able to:

1. Design meal plans for a balanced, low-calorie diet using food exchanges.

2. Specify key nutrition counseling strategies for weight control.

INTRODUCTION

Designing a balanced low-calorie diet that will promote gradual weight loss and teaching strategies for lifetime weight control are both difficult and rewarding. Using information obtained from the initial assessment, nurses can work as a team with other health professionals and the patient to develop an individualized weight control plan. There is no one single approach that works for all people. Any effective weight loss program must be tailored to each person's likes, dislikes, and lifestyle.

In most instances, a registered dietitian is available to assist with the initial dietary assessment and development of the weight control plan. As a member of the health care team, however, the nurse will often work with the dietitian to teach and implement this plan. If a registered dietitian is not available, the nurse may be called upon to help develop the weight loss plan. In either case, nurses must have an understanding of the basic principles of designing diet plans.

CHARACTERISTICS OF BALANCED WEIGHT LOSS DIETS

Many methods are used for weight control, including balanced low-calorie diets, very low-calorie diets, surgery, and drug therapy. Instruction in exercise and behavior modification can be combined with each of these therapies. Since balanced low-calorie dieting combined with exercise and behavior modification is the method appropriate for most overweight individuals, it is the one discussed here.

In designing and evaluating balanced low-calorie diet plans for weight loss, both safety and effectiveness must be considered. Since the ultimate goal of weight control efforts is long-term weight maintenance, weight loss approaches should build on principles of sound nutrition that can be carried into the weight maintenance phase.

Dwyer (1992) lists four characteristics of low-calorie diet plans:

1. The diet should provide a safe, calorie level.

2. The diet should be nutritionally balanced, with carbohydrate, protein, and fat provided in the right balance.

3. The overall weight loss plan should include other components essential to weight control, such as instruction in exercise and behavior modification.

4. The cost of the diet plan should be reasonable.

SAFE CALORIE LEVELS

One of the first steps in weight reduction is to establish the number of calories that will lead to a slow but sure loss of weight. Most successful weight-loss programs recommend that dieters try to reach a goal of losing 1 to 2 pounds per week. Although dieter and counselor alike may wish this loss were greater, it has been shown that successful dieters lose between 1.4 and 1.69 pounds per week. In the earliest stages of dieting, weight is lost more quickly. Diets that restrict calories to fewer than 1,200 per day may fail to provide enough nutrition. They may also lead to a physiological accommoda-

tion to the reduced food intake by a reduction in energy expended (Danish, 1968).

The difference between the calories expended and the calories ingested is called the *calorie deficit*. A calorie deficit of 3,500 will lead to the loss of 1 pound of body fat.

A patient can expect to lose about one pound per week with a calorie deficit of 500 calories per day (7 × 500 = 3,500 calories). A patient can expect to lose about two pounds per week with a calorie deficit of 1,000 calories per day (7 × 1,000 = 7,000 calories divided by 3,500 calories in a pound = 2 pounds). Since it is very difficult to exercise away 500 or more calories daily, the calorie deficit should ideally be obtained by a combination of cutting calories out of the diet and by increasing physical activity.

One way to determine a calorie level for weight loss is to use the initial dietary assessment. Current calorie intake can be estimated using food records or 24-hour food recalls for typical days. To lose weight, the patient must eat 500 to 1,000 calories less than is currently eaten daily, or achieve an equivalent calorie deficit by combining calorie reduction with increased physical activity.

Another approach is to estimate calories for weight maintenance using the following figures for varying activity levels:

- Sedentary: 10–12 calories per pound actual body weight
- Active: 13–15 calories per pound actual body weight
- Very active: 16–20 calories per pound of actual body weight

Then subtract 500 to 1,000 calories daily for weight loss.

Most inactive women maintain weight with about 1,600 to 1,800 calories daily. Most inactive men maintain weight with about 2,400 to 2,600 calories daily. (Men usually require more calories than women because they have more lean body mass, which burns more calories.) Therefore most women will lose about a pound a week on 1,200 calories daily, while most men will lose about a pound a week on 1,800 calories daily. If the individual also increases activity, weight loss will be greater.

Dwyer (1992) offers guidelines for selecting a safe, calorie level for weight loss:

- The calorie deficit should not exceed 1,000 calories without medical supervision.
- The diet should not be lower than 800 calories without medical supervision.
- For children, pregnant or lactating women, or individuals with illnesses or emotional difficulties who are trying to control weight, medical advice should be sought first.

Determining a calorie level for weight loss is always an estimate. Calorie levels may need adjusting on follow-up visits and as the individual loses weight. Also, patients differ in their ability to lose weight on a set calorie level because of differences in adherence, physical activity, body metabolism, diet composition, and water balance. Some individuals may also underestimate portion sizes or overestimate physical activity.

NUTRIENT COMPOSITION OF DIETS

Low-calorie diets should provide the right balance of carbohydrates, proteins, and fats. Nutritional recommendations for the general population are that carbohydrates should provide about 55 to 60 percent of total calories, fat should provide less than 30 percent of calories, and protein should provide 10 to 15 percent.

Fat is the most concentrated source of calories, so reducing fat in the diet will help dieters get a greater volume of food for fewer calories. Gram for gram, carbohydrates provide less than one-half the calories of fat, so foods rich in carbohydrates and fiber should be emphasized in a weight loss program.

Guidelines for appropriate nutrient composition of low-calorie diets are (Dwyer, 1992):

- 100 grams or more of carbohydrate, to spare body protein,
- A minimum of about 44 grams of high-quality protein for women and about 56 grams for men,
- Less than 30 percent of calories as fat,
- 20–30 grams of dietary fiber daily,
- Less than 200 milligrams of cholesterol daily,
- At least 1 liter of water daily, or 1 ml/calorie/day,
- An intake of vitamins and minerals at least equal to values specified by the Recommended Dietary Allowances (See Chapter 6).

As the calorie level of the diet decreases, the percentage of calories provided by protein will increase to achieve the minimum recommended level of protein daily. At calorie intakes of less than 1,200, it may be necessary to take a low-dose multivitamin and mineral preparation to achieve adequate intake of vitamins and minerals.

THE EXCHANGE LISTS FOR WEIGHT MANAGEMENT

To lose weight, some individuals may prefer to count daily calorie intake and follow the basic recommended number of servings from the food guide pyramid presented in Chapter 6. This approach is acceptable and teaches principles of sound nutrition for weight maintenance. Some individuals do not want to keep track of calories, others require a more structured diet.

Dietitians and other health care professionals have traditionally used exchange lists in designing individual meal plans for patients. The food exchange groups food with similar calorie and nutrient levels together, so one food can be substituted for another in each list. For example, a slice of bread and 1/2 cup of pasta are both on the starch/bread list. Each contains about 80 calories and similar amounts of carbohydrates, vitamins, proteins, and other essential nutrients.

The American Diabetes and Dietetic Associations jointly released the latest Food Exchange Lists for Weight Management (1989). A simplified, pictorial version of these exchange lists called *Eating Healthy Foods* is also available and is especially useful for patients with limited reading skills (The American Diabetes Association and The American Dietetic Association, 1988).

The exchange lists divide foods into six groups: starch/bread, meat, vegetable, fruit, milk, and fat. Nurses or dietitians can specify the number of servings a patient should have from each exchange list daily. The approximate calorie and nutrient composition of the diet will be known without the patient having to keep track of calories.

The size of a portion is important, and each serving is one exchange. If the portion is doubled, it equals 2 exchanges. For example, two slices of whole wheat bread equal two bread exchanges. For example: 1 bread exchange = 1 slice of bread or 1 small potato or 1/2 cup cooked cereal.

Exchange lists are an easy way to plan nutritious, sensible, and interesting meals. Most of the lists contain very common foods. Foods can be exchanged or substituted for each other only in the same exchange group.

The foods in each of the six exchange lists are summarized in Table 7.1. Table 7.2 gives the calorie and nutrient content in each of the six groups.

STEPS IN CALCULATING A MEAL PLAN

Calculating meal plans based on the exchange lists can be simplified by following the steps listed below:

1. Estimate energy needs for maintenance and subtract 500 to 1,000 calories, with 1,000 calories the lowest limit.

2. Distribute calories into desired percentages of protein, carbohydrate, and fat. For example, for a diet that supplies 20 percent of calories as protein, 55 percent as carbohydrate, and 25 percent as fat, multiply calorie level by 0.20 for protein, 0.55 for carbohydrate, and 0.25 for fat.

3. Convert calories from protein, carbohydrate, and fat into grams by dividing protein calories by 4 calories per gram, carbohydrate, calories by 4 calories per gram, and fat calories by 9 calories per gram.

Table 7.1 Exchange List Summary Sheet

For all MEAT/PROTEIN CHOICES, 1 Exchange = 1 ounce or amount indicated, cooked, boneless, and skinless

LOW-FAT MEAT/PROTEIN CHOICES
Beef:
   Flank steak, London broil, round steak
Poultry:
   Chicken, Cornish hen, turkey
Fish:
   Halibut; red snapper; water-packed salmon or tuna, 1/4 cup; shrimp, 2 oz.
Cheese:
   Low-fat/2% cottage cheese, 1/4 cup; grated Parmesan, 2 Tbsp.; diet cheeses with 55 Calories or less per ounce
Other:
   Dried beans and peas, cooked, 1/2 cup (count 1/2 Bread/Starch)

MEDIUM-FAT MEAT/PROTEIN CHOICES
COUNT 1/2 FAT FOR EACH EXCHANGE
Beef:
   Pot roast, groundbeef or ground round (85% lean),rump roast
Lamb:
   Leg roast, loin chop
Pork:
   Sirloin, chop, loin roast
Cheeses:
   Part-skim mozzarella;part-skim ricotta, 1/4 cup.
   Neufchatel, 2 Tbsp.
Egg,
   1 whole
Luncheon Meats/Sausages:
   Chicken roll, turkey bologna
Other:
   Peanut butter, 1 Tbsp.

HIGH-FAT MEAT/PROTEIN CHOICES
COUNT 1 FAT FOR EACH EXCHANGE
Beef:
   Brisket, hamburger (80% lean or less), sirloin steak
Pork:
   Ribs, country style/spareribs
Cheeses:
   American, Cheddar, Swiss
Luncheon Meats/Sausages
   Beef and pork bologna, salami, bratwurst, Spam, frankfurters

BREAD/STARCH CHOICES
Bread, 1 slice
Pita or pocket bread, 1/2 of 6" diameter
Roll, 1 - 2" across
Tortilla, 1 - 6" diameter corn (unfried)
Starchy Vegetables:
   Corn on the cob, 6"
   Green peas, 1/2 cup
   White potato, 1/2 cup
   Yam or sweet potato, plain,1/3 cup
Cereals:
   Cooked (oats, farina, etc.),1/2 cup
   Flake, 3/4 cup
Grains:
   Macaroni or pasta, plain cooked, 1/2 cup
   Rice, white or brown, plain cooked, 1/3 cup
Crackers and Snacks:
   Popcorn, plain popped, 3 cups
   Ritz-type crackers, 6 (count 1 Fat)
   Saltines, 6 - 2" square
   Wheat Thins, 12 (count 1 Fat)
Desserts:
   Graham crackers, 3 - 2 1/2" square
   Ice cream, 1/2 cup (count 2 Fat)
   Sherbet, 1/4 cup

MILK CHOICES
Skim/nonfat milk or yogurt, 1 cup
Low-fat milk or yogurt, 1 cup (count 1 Fat)
Whole milk or yogurt, 1 cup (count 1 1/2 Fat)

FREE CHOICES
When consumed in small amounts, these items have few Calories and little sugar or fat
Beverages
   Club soda, coffee, tea
Sauces/Relishes/Seasonings:
   Horseradish, vinegar, flavoring extracts, herbs, lemon juice (unsweetened)

VEGETABLE CHOICES
1/2 cup cooked or 1 cup raw or amount indicated of these vegetables alone or mixed:
Green beans, beets;
broccoli, carrots; eggplant;
jicama, onions, tomato, 1 medium;
tomato sauce, 3 Tbsp

These items can be eaten freely, their Calorie content is especially low
Cucumber, lettuce, mushrooms, green onions or scallions, peppers, radishes, spinach, zucchini

FRUIT
Apple, 1 - 2" diameter
Banana, 1/2 of 9" long
Berries:
   Blueberries, 3/4 cup
   Strawberries, 1 1/4 cup
Grapes, 15 small
Melon:
   Cantaloupe, 1/3 of 5" diameter
   Watermelon, 1 1/4 cups cubed
Orange, 1 small
Pear, 1 small
Raisins, 2 Tbsp.
Juices
   Apple juice/cider, 1/2 cup
   Cranberry cocktail (regular), 1/3 cup
   Grape juice, 1/3 cup
   Grapefruit juice, 1/2 cup
   Orange juice, 1/2 cup
   Peach nectar, 1/3 cup
   Pineapple juice, 1/2 cup

FAT CHOICES
Avocado, 1/8 of 4" across
Bacon, 1 strip
Butter or margarine, 1 tsp
Margarine, diet or whipped, 1 Tbsp.
Oil or shortening, 1 tsp.
Cream cheese, 1 Tbsp.
Cream, light or half & half, 2 Tbsp.
Mayonnaise, 1 tsp.
Olives, green or black, 10 small
Nuts:
   Almonds, 6
   Peanuts, 10 large
   Walnuts, 4 halves
Salad Dressings
   Bleu cheese/Roquefort, 2 tsp.
   Italian or vinegar & oil, 1 Tbsp.

Source: The American Dietetic Association, The American Diabetes Association. *Exchange Lists for Weight Management* 1989.

Table 7.2 Nutrients in Grams and Calories

Exchange List	Carbohydrate (grams)	Protein (grams)	Fat (grams)	Calories
Starch/Bread	15	3	trace	80
Meat				
Lean	–	7	3	55
Medium-Fat	–	7	5	75
High-Fat	–	7	8	100
Vegetable	5	2	–	25
Fruit	15	–	–	60
Milk				
Skim	12	8	trace	90
Lowfat	12	8	5	120
Whole	12	8	8	150
Fat	–	–	5	45

Source: The American Dietetic Association, The American Diabetes Association, *Exchange Lists for Weight Management,* 1989.

4. Translate grams of protein, carbohydrate, and fat into exchanges from the food list. Pick the number of servings from each exchange group according to individual food preferences. Add up grams of protein, carbohydrate, and fat from each exchange group and adjust number of servings as needed to approximate desired grams of protein, carbohydrate, and fat.

5. Distribute the servings from all the exchange lists into meals and snacks based on the individual's usual dietary habits. Individuals taking insulin will need to have their exchanges distributed to match insulin schedules as well as food preferences.

SAMPLE MEAL PLANS

A Sample 1,200-calorie Meal Plan

To design a meal plan for an inactive, middle-aged female who weighs 170 pounds:

1. *Estimate energy needs.* An estimate of her calorie needs to maintain weight would be 170 pounds × 10 calories per pound = 1,700 calories. To lose about a pound weekly, subtract 500 calories daily, leaving a calorie level for weight loss of 1,200 calories daily. (You will also help the patient work out an exercise plan, which should help her lose more than a pound weekly.)

2. *Distribute calories.*
   carbohydrate: 0.55 × 1.200 calories = 660 calories
   protein: 0.20 × 1.200 calories = 240 calories
   fat: 0.25 × 1.200 calories = 300 calories

3. *Convert calories to grams.*

660 calories ÷ 4 calories per gram = 165 grams of carbohydrate

240 calories ÷ 4 calories per gram = 60 grams of protein

300 calories ÷ 9 calories per gram = 33 grams of fat

4. *Translate grams into exchanges.*

When translating grams of nutrients into exchange groups, keep the individual's usually dietary pattern in mind. The greater the calorie level of the diet, the more flexibility you have in planning the exchanges. The following meal plan would provide approximately the desired calories and grams of carbohydrate, protein, and fat:

6 starch/bread exchanges

4 lean meat exchanges

3 vegetable exchanges

2 fruit exchanges

2 skim milk exchanges

3 fat exchanges

5. *Distribute exchanges into meals and snacks.* Again, it is helpful to base distribution of exchanges on the individual's usual eating pattern, unless the patient must follow a more rigid meal pattern because of insulin or other medication use. If a patient is accustomed to having several snacks daily, then plan them into the meal pattern. However, avoid consumption of the bulk of the exchanges late in the day.

It is also helpful to give patients a sample menu.

Breakfast:

2 starch/bread exchange	1 ounce ready-to-eat cereal
	1 slice whole-grain toast
1 fat exchange	1 teaspoon margarine
1 milk exchange	1 cup skim milk
1 fruit exchange	1/2 grapefruit

Lunch:

1 starch/bread exchange	2 slices pumpernickel
1 meat exchange	1 ounce sliced turkey

1 fat exchange	1 tablespoon reduced-calorie mayonnaise
free food	lettuce
1 fruit exchange	1 1/4 cut whole strawberries
1 vegetable exchange	1 cup raw carrot sticks

Supper:

3 meat exchanges	6 ounces boiled shrimp
1 starch exchange	1 small baked potato
2 vegetable exchanges	1 cup cooked broccoli
1 fat exchange	1 teaspoon margarine
free food	decaffeinated coffee

Snack:

1 milk exchange	8 ounces plain non-fat yogurt
1 starch/bread exchange	3 graham cracker squares

A Sample 1,800-calorie Meal Plan

Following the same steps as listed above, this 1,800-calorie meal plan was developed:

9 starch/bread exchanges

3 lean meat exchanges

3 medium-fat meat exchanges

3 vegetable exchanges

3 fruit exchanges

2 skim milk exchanges

5 fat exchanges

NUTRITION COUNSELING SKILLS

For nutrition counseling to be most effective, nutrition counselors should:

• Create a good setting.

• Build rapport using good communication.

• Listen carefully.

• Avoid yes and no questions.

• Help the patient identify and plan goals.

• Give frequent feedback.

• Be specific about what is expected.

• Encourage family involvement.

• Be supportive.

The next chapter will give some specific advice on implementing weight loss diets in a variety of settings. Tips for keeping food diaries, grocery shopping, reading labels, cooking meals, planning, and eating out will be given.

EXAM QUESTIONS

Chapter 7

Questions 59-66

59. What member of the health care team usually provides valuable assistance in designing diet plans?

    a. licensed nutritionist
    b. exercise physiologist
    c. physician
    d. registered dietitian

60. Balanced, low-calorie diets should provide what percentage of total calorie intake from carbohydrates?

    a. 35-40%
    b. 45-50%
    c. 55-60%
    d. 65-70%

61. Which of the following is not a characteristic of effective low-calorie weight loss plans:

    a. safe calorie level
    b. nutritionally balanced diet
    c. includes other components such as exercise and behavior modification
    d. drug therapy

62. Sedentary individuals usually maintain body weight on how many calories per pound of actual body weight?

    a. 16-20
    b. 13-15
    c. 10-12
    d. 7-9

63. By cutting 500 calories from the daily diet, a person can expect a weekly weight loss of:

    a. 1 pound
    b. 2 pounds
    c. 3 pounds
    d. 0.5 pound

64. Most women will lose about one pound weekly on how many calories daily?

    a. 800
    b. 1,200
    c. 1,500
    d. 1,800

65. Which food exchange list do potatoes belong in?

    a. starch/bread list
    b. vegetable list
    c. fat list
    d. combination list

66. In designing meal plans, the first step is to:

    a. distribute calories
    b. translate protein, carbohydrate, and fat into exchanges
    c. determine percentage of protein, carbohydrate, and fat
    d. estimate energy needs for weight maintenance

CHAPTER 8

DIET INTERVENTION
IMPLEMENTING DIET PLANS

CHAPTER OBJECTIVE

After reading this chapter, you will be able to describe food-related behaviors and activities that can improve adherence to diet plans.

LEARNING OBJECTIVES

After studying this chapter, you will be able to:

1. Identify advantages of keeping a food diary.

2. Describe aspects of cooking, menu planning, grocery shopping, label reading, and eating out that promote weight loss and maintenance.

3. Select strategies that enhance patient motivation.

INTRODUCTION

Knowing what to do and doing it are very different actions. Often a patient will understand that he or she needs to reduce calories and eat less fat, but

will have difficulty doing so. Giving specific and practical advice about food-related activities and behaviors will help patients bridge the gap between knowing what to do, and doing it. This chapter will give practical suggestions on food diaries, meal planning, grocery shopping, label reading, and eating out to enhance patient adherence to diet plans. Suggestions to help motivate patients to action are also given.

KEEPING A FOOD DIARY

Having patients keep a daily food diary usually improves adherence to recommended diet changes. At each visit to the nurse, dietitian, or other health professional, the diet diary can be reviewed for adherence and provide a teaching tool. Keeping a daily food diary accomplishes several goals:

- Increases awareness of food intake.
- Provides a teaching tool to learn about aspects of the diet or calorie content of foods.
- Helps patients and counselors learn about eating patterns and relationship of eating to other events or feelings.
- Fosters control over eating.
- Provides a written record of calories, which can be related to weight change.

Date _____   Name _____

Time		Place	Phy Pos	Alone or with whom	Assoc. Activity	M	H	M / S	Amount	Food or Beverage	Calories
Start	End										
6-11											
11-4											
4-9											
9-6											

Percent of entries filled out right before or after eating   0   25   50   75   100

Figure 8.1 Food intake record.

Source: Henry A. Jordan, Leonard S. Levitz, and Gordon M. Kimbrell, "Food Intake Record" from *Eating Is Okay*. Copyright© 1976 by Associates for Behavioral Education and S & R Gelman Associates Inc. Reprinted with permission of Rawson Associates; an imprint of Macmillian Publishing Company.

Figure 8.1 shows a sample of a very detailed food diary where the patient records not only the type and amount of food eaten, but also the time the patient started and stopped eating, the place, the physical position, whom the patient was with, what the patient was doing while eating, the patient's mood, the patient's hunger level at the time, and whether the food was considered a meal or snack.

Detailed diaries such as this are often used in behavior modification programs. Diaries help patients and counselors learn about behaviors, emotions, and activities that promote overeating and weight gain. However, it is not always necessary for patients to keep such detailed diaries. Even a simple record of food or drink and amount scratched daily on a pocket notebook will greatly increase patient awareness of diet and improve diet adherence. If the patient has an exercise prescription, he or she may also want to record that on the daily food diary.

For the greatest effectiveness, patients should be instructed to record *everything* they eat or drink, except for water. They should record this right after eating, not later that evening or the next day. To do this, the food diary should be carried with the patient wherever he or she goes.

PLANNING MENUS

Nurses and dietitians should encourage patients to plan their meals and snacks ahead of time. When meals and snacks are planned ahead, the patient is more likely to make food selections consistent with his or her diet plan and less likely to eat on impulse. When meals and snacks are preplanned, the patient knows what the next meal is going to be, can start fixing it in a timely manner, and can have the right ingredients on hand. The patient is less likely to eat whatever comes to mind or sight. Preplanning also allows patients to have nutritious, low-calorie snacks available and to keep problem foods out of the house.

Patients vary widely in the amount of preplanning they do. The counselor should assess the current level of preplanning and encourage the patient to plan more. Some patients plan from meal to meal. In this case, encourage them to plan from day to day. Some patients plan one day at a time and can be encouraged to plan a week at a time. If certain meals pose problems in terms of fat and calorie content, work on planning these first. For example, breakfast and lunch might be fairly straightforward;

all that really needs to be planned are the evening meals.

The time it takes to sit down and preplan meals and snacks will be saved by more efficient grocery shopping, simpler meal preparation, and greater diet adherence.

PREPARING FOOD

Since 70 percent of the calorie intake of Americans comes from foods prepared at home, focusing on low-fat cooking methods yields a large payoff in terms of calorie savings. Some weight loss courses include cooking demonstrations.

Diet counselors must also remember that many Americans are pressed for time and do not want to bother with time-consuming yet healthy recipes. A recent survey noted that 40 percent of Americans don't like the way they eat but think it's too much work to change. Fortunately, many healthy, low-fat foods require little preparation. Fresh fruits, vegetables, and breads are readily available and easy to prepare.

Here are some tips to reduce calories and fat in food preparation and menu planning:

Meat, Poultry, and Fish
- Grill, bake, broil, or boil instead of fry.
- Trim off all visible fat and remove skin from poultry before cooking.
- Drain meat frequently while cooking.
- Choose leaner cuts of meat.
- Marinade less tender meats in vinegar or wine before cooking.

Dairy Products
- Use skim milk in soups, puddings, and baked products.

- Substitute skimmed milk for evaporated milk in recipes.
- Substitute low-fat cottage cheese or yogurt for sour cream.

Grains

- Use jelly or jam instead of butter on toast.
- Choose hard rolls, bagels, English muffins, or yeast breads in place of sweet rolls, doughnuts, or biscuits.
- Use pasta, rice, or other grains in casseroles and mixed dishes to increase carbohydrate content and decrease fat content.

Vegetables

- Microwave or steam vegetables until just crisp and tender.
- Learn to enjoy the natural flavor of vegetables and avoid adding butter or sauce.
- Eat salads with lemon, vinegar, or non-fat dressings.

Fruit

- Try less common fruits like fresh berries, fresh pineapple, or kiwi fruit for a special treat.
- Eat fresh fruit for dessert.

GROCERY SHOPPING

Grocery shopping is a critical point of control for individuals trying to lose or maintain weight. A typical grocery store contains thousands of foods. Diet counselors should emphasize that the food purchased is the food that will be eaten. If the patient wants to limit or avoid certain foods, they shouldn't be brought into the house. If the patient wants to eat more fruits, vegetables, and whole grains, these are the foods that should be purchased.

Many fresh fruits and vegetables remain fairly inexpensive all year long. If time is a factor, cut or sliced foods are worth the additional cost. Many stores sell washed and cut fresh vegetables and boneless, skinless meats. Several lines of low-calorie frozen dinners are also available. Patients should be encouraged to select dinners that contain 300 calories or less and 10 grams of fat or less. Patients will also need instruction on rounding out the nutrient content of frozen dinners with fresh fruits, vegetables, and non-fat dairy products.

Suggest that the patient preplan meals and shop from a grocery list. Shopping from a list helps reduce impulse buying. Also suggest that the patient avoid shopping when hungry or tired. When shopping, encourage the patient to stock up on these foods:

- rice
- pasta
- dried or canned beans and peas
- fresh fruits and vegetables
- fruits canned in juice or water
- frozen vegetables or low-salt canned vegetables
- 100 percent fruit juice
- diet salad dressing
- fish
- chicken, turkey, or game hens
- lean red meat such as beef round, loin, sirloin, flank, and extra lean ground beef; pork tenderloin, leg, shoulder, and ham; or leg, arm, loin and rib of lamb
- lean deli meats
- skim milk
- non-fat yogurt
- low-fat cheese
- popcorn
- water-packed tuna
- rice cakes
- whole-grain breads and rolls
- whole-grain breakfast cereals
- graham or soda crackers
- broth-based soups

READING LABELS

Following the National Nutrition Labeling and Education Act of 1990, a major overhaul of the food labeling system took place. New laws now require labels on virtually all foods. Patients should be encouraged to study labels, particularly for information on type of fat, fat content, and calorie content.

Consider the sample food label shown in Figure 8.2. The amount of calories in a serving and calories from fat are clearly indicated at the top of the label. By dividing fat calories by total calories, patients can easily figure the percentage of calories that come from fat in a particular food. Using Figure 8.2 as an example, 120 fat calories divided by 260 total calories multiplied by 100% means that 46 percent of this food's calories come from fat.

A reasonable dietary goal is to keep intake of fat to less than 30 percent of daily calories. This does not mean that every food a patient eats must contain less than 30 percent of calories from fat. If a patients eats foods with a higher fat content, they must be balanced with foods of lower fat content.

Before the new labeling regulations, some food manufacturers made questionable health claims for products or used terms like "light" or "low." Under the new regulations, only well-substantiated health claims are allowed on packages, and descriptors like "free," "low," "lean," "extra lean," "high," "good source," "reduced," "less," "light," and "more" have specific definitions.

With regard to calorie content, "low" means less than 40 calories. "Reduced" means that the product contains 25 percent fewer calories than the regular food. "Light" means that the product contains one-third fewer calories than the regular food.

EATING OUT

The average American spends 40 cents of every food dollar away from home, of this, 16 cents at fast food restaurants. Individuals trying to lose or maintain weight can easily eat out if they plan ahead, learn to ask questions, make special requests, and emphasize the same types of foods at restaurants as they do at home. Since it is the overall balance of the diet that is important, the more often patients eat out, the more important their selections at restaurants become.

In keeping with the increased health awareness, most restaurants offer at least a few healthy choices on their menus. At fast-food restaurants, the plain sandwiches or hamburgers usually contain the fewest calories (see Appendix B for a list of calorie and fat content of some fast foods). Many fast-food restaurants also offer salads, but if you add in the calories in the large packet of dressing, a burger might be a better choice.

At a full service restaurant, choose fresh breads or rolls, pasta and rice dishes, and vegetables. Patients might order a fresh fruit cup to complement their meal. Italian, Mexican, seafood, and Chinese restaurants are some of the types of restaurants where several lower-calories selections are available.

Patients should also learn to ask questions about how food is prepared and make special requests. Patients can ask that the fish be broiled without added fat, that the butter be left off the vegetables, or that sauces be served on the side.

At a vending machine, patients should be encouraged to choose plain yogurt, a piece of fruit, fruit juice, or crackers. With microwaves available at many work sites, brown bag lunches can be an extension of home-cooked foods, with soups, stews, casseroles, and salads some of the many choices.

Serving sizes are more consistent across product lines.

New title signals the newly required information.

Nutrition Facts

Serving Size 1/2 cup (114g)
Servings Per Container 4

Amount Per Serving

Calories 90   Calories from Fat 30

Calories from fat are shown to help consumers meet dietary guidelines.

% **Daily Value***

The list of nutrients covers those most important to the health of today's consumers.

Total Fat 3g	**5**%
Saturated Fat 0g	**0**%
Cholesterol 0mg	**0**%
Sodium 300mg	**13**%
Total Carbohydrate 13g	**4**%
Dietary Fiber 3g	**12**%
Sugars 3g	
Protein 3g	

%Daily Value shows how a food fits into the overall daily diet.

Vitamin A	80%	Vitamin C	60%
Calcium	4%	Iron	4%

* Percent Daily Values are based on a 2.000 calorie diet. Your daily values may be higher or lower depending on your calorie needs:

		Calories	2000	2500
Total Fat	Less than		65g	80g
Sat Fat	Less than		20g	25g
Cholesterol	Less than		300mg	300mg
Sodium	Less than		2400mg	2400mg
Total Carbohydrate			300g	375g
Fiber			25g	30g

Calories per gram:
Fat 9   •   Carbohydrates 4   •   Protein 4

The label tells the number of calories per gram of fat, carbohydrates and protein.

The daily values on the label are based on a daily diet of 2000 and 2500 calories.

Figure 8.2 The new food label.

Source: FDA Press Kit, Jan 1992.

When traveling by air, call at least 24 hours ahead of departure to ask about heart-healthy or light meals. They often consist of seafood or fruit platters and are often very appealing. When staying in a hotel, take along some food. Small boxes of breakfast cereal, instant oatmeal, and fresh fruit travel well.

STRATEGIES TO ENHANCE PATIENT ADHERENCE

The National Heart, Lung, and Blood Institute (1991) gives eight tips to help improve patient adherence to diet plans:

1. *Relate* If nurses can relate well with their patients and develop a close and caring relationship, the patient will be more likely to adhere to advice given.

2. *Communicate* Be clear in what you are trying to say. Give specific advice, repeat it, and ask the patient to repeat it to be certain they understand what you are saying.

3. *Motivate* Increase motivation by reducing diet changes into small, progressive steps, and setting realistic short-term goals.

4. *Educate* Use or develop educational aids to help patients understand their current eating patterns and the desired eating patterns.

5. *Collaborate* Encourage support from the patient's family and refer the patient to other professionals or self-help or support groups as needed.

6. *Facilitate* Make dietary changes easier by making changes gradually. Keep changes as simple as possible.

7. *Innovate* Use innovative methods to increase adherence, such as giving token rewards for short-term goals achieved, having patients contribute their favorite healthy recipes, or creating a lending library of related health or cookbooks.

8. *Calculate* Keep track of the success of your patients in reaching diet, exercise, and weight loss goals. Note improvements in blood pressure, blood cholesterol levels, blood sugar levels, and other risk factors for chronic diseases.

Certain groups of patients need special dietary consideration. The next chapter will discuss nutritional concerns for individuals with or at risk for diabetes, cardiovascular disease, high blood pressure, and cancer. The chapter will also present some special considerations for both young and old patients.

EXAM QUESTIONS

Chapter 8

Questions 67-74

67. In planning menus, which types of foods should be emphasized overall?

    a. quick and convenient foods
    b. protein foods
    c. diet dressings and spreads
    d. breads and rolls

68. What percentage of calories do Americans get from foods prepared at home?

    a. 40%
    b. 55%
    c. 70%
    d. 95%

69. Which tool is frequently used to increase eating awareness?

    a. waist cord
    b. food diary
    c. food frequency questionnaire
    d. jaw wire

70. Using the new food label, patients can determine percentage of calories from fat in a food by:

    a. dividing fat calories by total calories
    b. multiplying the grams of fat by 9
    c. dividing grams of fat by total calories
    d. this cannot be determined from the new food label

71. Obese individuals should be encouraged to:

    a. shop for groceries as infrequently as possible
    b. shop when the store is busy
    c. avoid grocery shopping if at all possible
    d. shop from a planned list

72. How many cents out of every food dollar does the average American spend away from home?

    a. $0.20
    b. $0.30
    c. $0.40
    d. $0.50

73. Under the new labeling regulations, food manufacturers can use terms like "low" and "reduced":

    a. in an unrestricted manner
    b. only if they apply for permission first
    c. food manufacturers can no longer use such terms
    d. only if their products meet the strict definitions for these terms

74. For an individual trying to lose weight, which of the following would probably be the best choice at a fast food restaurant?

    a. a plain burger
    b. a salad with dressing
    c. a baked potato with cheese
    d. a fish sandwich

CHAPTER 9

DIET INTERVENTION
FOR SPECIAL POPULATIONS

CHAPTER OBJECTIVE

After reading this chapter, you will be able to identify dietary considerations for special groups of patients.

LEARNING OBJECTIVES

After studying this chapter, you will be able to:

1. Discuss specific dietary guidelines for treatment or prevention of diabetes, atherosclerosis, high blood pressure, and cancer.

2. Specify dietary considerations for young and elderly patients.

INTRODUCTION

In addition to helping healthy, overweight patients, nurses may help overweight patients with certain diseases or special nutritional needs. Such groups of people include those with cardiovascular disease, high blood lipid levels, high blood pressure, or type I or II diabetes. Elderly individuals, children, adolescents, and individuals concerned about or at risk for cancer may also require special dietary considerations.

DIABETES

Nearly 11 million Americans have diabetes. By far the majority — about 85 percent — have non-insulin-dependent diabetes (Grundy, 1987). Complications from diabetes make it the fifth leading cause of death in our country.

Obesity is a substantial risk factor for type II diabetes, the kind of diabetes that usually occurs later in life (Riccardo, 1992). About 80 percent of individuals with type II diabetes are obese. Obesity aggravates diabetes by raising blood sugar levels and increasing insulin resistance. Weight loss usually decreases the need for medication or insulin in type II diabetes and may even reverse the disease.

Ironically, diabetes may be a genetic modification that once served as a superior survival trait. Researchers such as Graber theorize that diabetes was once a "thrifty gene" trait that provided better storage and metabolism of food when food was hard to obtain and store (1977). As food became more plentiful, the negative parts of the trait emerged.

The Pima Indians of the Gila and Salt River areas in southern Arizona have provided a good example of the effect of the "thrifty gene" trait (National Center for Health Statistics, 1986). The Pimas lived in an arid, desolate land, where it was very difficult to meet nutritional needs. Today, after adopting the lifestyles and diets of typical suburban Americans, the Pimas have a greater than normal tendency to be obese. In additon, nearly half of the adults have developed diabetes.

Weight loss is a primary goal for obese individuals with type II diabetes, along with maintaining normal blood glucose and lipid levels. A diabetic diet is designed to help patients lose weight and bring their weight under control by reducing the consumption of fats and sugar (American Diabetes Association, 1992). Many diabetics are at risk of atherosclerosis, resulting in heart attacks and stroke. It is important that both a low-calorie and a low-fat diet be used. There are people who are at risk of developing the disease even if they control their weight.

It is essential to tailor-make diets for individual patients, so that the needs, abilities, and resources of the individual are met. With these patients, reinforcement and encouragement are usually necessary for the dietary program to succeed. Treatment of diabetes involves attaining ideal body weight. An obese person must take in fewer calories than are expended. The nutritional needs for diabetic patients are not different from those for other patients, so the RDA guidelines can be used for planning and evaluating diabetic diets. Diets low in fat are particularly important, since degenerative vascular changes occur far more rapidly in diabetic than in nondiabetic persons (American Heart Association, 1987).

The type of carbohydrate consumed is also important. Insulin is given so that it reaches its peak concentration in the blood at the same time the blood sugar level reaches its highest level. It is also given in a dose designed to bring the blood sugar back to normal without producing hypoglycemia. A consistent eating pattern is important. The patient must try to consume the same number of calories at every meal, and every snack, at approximately the same time every day. By manipulating the foods and snacks, the diet can be adjusted to fit the individual's lifestyle and needs (American Diabetes Association, 1992).

In recent times, dietary fiber has received quite a bit of attention. Several studies have shown that increasing dietary fiber intake, particularly soluble fiber, reduces blood sugar levels, blood lipid levels, and insulin requirements (Anderson, 1987). The American Diabetes Association (1992) recommends that fiber intake be gradually increased to a maximum total of 40 grams of fiber daily, or 25 grams per 1000 calories.

The glycemic index is another important dietary measure for diabetic persons. This is a means of measuring the speed at which different foods raise blood-sugar levels. Glucose is given a value of 100. Other foods are then related to it and to each other as a percentage of the absorption of glucose. The number assigned to each food is the *glycemic index*. The lower the number, the more slowly the food raises the blood sugar. Here are some examples of foods and their glycemic indexes:

	(%)
White bread	69
Pastry	59
Oatmeal cookie	54
Carrots	92
Orange	40
Green beans	31
Cornflakes	80
Ice cream	36
Instant potato	80
New potato	70
Sweet potato	48
Potato chips	51

| Mars Bar | 68 |
| Sucrose, or refined sugar | 59 |

These findings make it appear that certain foods previously thought to affect the blood sugar very slowly actually have a higher glycemic index than refined sugar. Foods such as carrots, potatoes, and some cereals and breads fall into this category. Naturally, much study remains to be done to identify foods that rapidly raise the serum glucose level. The studies were done in a laboratory setting, not typical of our daily lives. Meals and mixtures of foods may vary widely, and foods may interact.

The exchange lists given in Chapter 7 are used to design diets for overweight diabetic individuals. Here are a few general guidelines for devising a diabetic diet (American Diabetes Association, 1992):

- Calories should be reduced so that the person can achieve ideal weight.

- Fats should make up only 20 to 30 percent of the total calories consumed.

- Saturated fats should supply 10 to 15 percent of the total calories, and polyunsaturated and monounsaturated fat, from vegetable sources, should provide the other 10 to 15 percent.

- Protein can make up from 12 to 24 percent of all calories, although these are only guidelines and aren't critical.

- Carbohydrates should provide 55 to 60 percent of total calories, with simple sugars restricted to 10 to 15 percent of all calories consumed.

- Cholesterol intake should be less than 300mg daily.

- Total dietary fiber intake should be 25 grams per 1000 calories.

ATHEROSCLEROSIS

Fear of the number-one cause of death in the United States, heart disease, has been a powerful motivator for many Americans to modify their diet. Obesity, particularly abdominal obesity, increases the risk of atherosclerotic cardiovascular disease both independently and through its effects on blood pressure, blood lipids, and blood glucose levels (Bierman, 1992).

High blood cholesterol levels, especially high levels of low-density lipoprotein (LDL) cholesterol, are associated with greater risk of coronary heart disease (CHD). Another type of lipoprotein, high-density lipoprotein (HDL) cholesterol, helps protect against CHD. The risk for CHD rises progressively with blood cholesterol levels above 200mg/dl. Risk sharply rises with cholesterol levels above 220mg/dl.

According to guidelines of the National Cholesterol Education Program of the National Institutes of Health (1989), a desirable blood cholesterol level for all adults is below 200mg/dl. A level between 200 and 239mg/dl is considered borderline high, and a level of 240mg/dl or greater is considered high.

All individuals should be given preventative diet information to reduce risk of heart disease. Obese individuals at risk for heart disease need to lose weight and lower total fat, saturated fat, and cholesterol content of their diet. These diet goals should also be actively pursued by individuals who have already experienced a heart attack (Rossouw, 1990).

For individuals with borderline high or high blood cholesterol levels, diet therapy and exercise is the first line of treatment, followed by a combination of diet and drug therapy if response to diet therapy is inadequate after six months (or sooner if lipids are severely elevated). Diet therapy can be implemented in a two-step fashion.

The "Step-One Diet" advocated by the National Cholesterol Education Program contains less than 30 percent of calories from fat, less than 10 percent of calories from saturated fat, and less than 300mg of dietary cholesterol per day. The "Step-Two Diet" goes a little farther by limiting saturated fat intake to 7 percent of calories and limiting dietary cholesterol to 200mg per day. The Step-Two Diet is used when response to the Step-One Diet is inadequate.

Most of the changes in the Step-One Diet can be made without drastically altering dietary patterns. The Step-Two Diet will require more careful attention to food selection. Table 9.1 outlines both step diets. Recommended diet modifications for the Step-One Diet are shown in Table 9.2. These diets for lowering serum lipid levels are very similar to recommendations of the American Heart Associa-

tion (1987). The American Heart Association also recommends limiting sodium intake to 130mEq daily.

The American Heart Association gives suggestions for limiting fat and cholesterol in the diet:

1. Read labels carefully. Foods made with vegetable oils, particularly palm and coconut oil, can still carry high percentages of saturated fats.

2. Chicken and turkey skin should be removed before cooking; most of the fat is in the skin.

3. All visible fat should be removed before cooking, and meats should be cooked in such a way that fat can drip away from the meat; meat drippings should be discarded.

Table 9.1 Dietary Therapy of High Blood Cholesterol

Nutrient	Recommended Intake	
	Step-One Diet	Step-Two Diet
Total Fat	Less than 30% of Total Calories	
Saturated Fatty Acids	Less than 10% of Total Calories	Less than 7% of Total Calories
Polyunsaturated Fatty Acids	Up to 10% of Total Calories	
Monounsaturated Fatty Acids	10 to 15% of Total Calories	
Carbohydrates	50 to 60% of Total Calories	
Protein	10 to 20% of Total Calories	
Cholesterol	Less than 300mg/day	Less than 200 mg/day
Total Calories	To achieve and maintain desirable weight	

Source: National Cholesterol Education Program. (1989). *Report of the Expert Panel on Detection, Evaluation, and Treatment of High Blood Cholesterol in Adults.* U.S. Department of Health and Human Services, Public Health Service, National Institutes of Health. NIH publication No. 89–2925. p. 30.

Table 9.2 Recommended Diet Modifications to Lower Blood Cholesterol: The Step-One Diet

	Choose	Decrease
Fish, Chicken, Turkey, and Lean Meats	Fish, poultry without skin, lean cuts of beef, lamb, pork or veal, shellfish	Fatty cuts of beef, lamb, pork; spare ribs, organ meats, regular cold cuts, sausage, hot dogs, bacon, sardines, roe
Skim and Low-Fat Milk, Cheese, Yogurt, and Dairy Substitutes	Skim or 1% fat milk (liquid, powdered, evaporated) Buttermilk	Whole milk (4% fat): regular, evaporated, condensed; cream, half and half, 2% milk, imitation milk products, most nondairy creamers, whipped toppings
	Nonfat (0% fat) or low-fat yogurt	Whole-milk yogurt
	Low-fat cottage cheese (1% or 2% fat)	Whole-milk cottage cheese (4% fat)
	Low-fat cheeses, farmer, or pot cheeses (all of these should be labeled no more than 2–6 g fat/ounce)	All natural cheeses (e.g. blue, roquefort, camembert, cheddar, swiss)
	Sherbet Sorbet	Low-fat or "light" cream cheese, low-fat or "light" sour cream
		Cream cheeses, sour cream
		Ice Cream
Eggs	Egg whites (2 whites=1 whole egg in recipes), cholesterol-free egg substitutes	Egg yolks
Fruits and Vegetables	Fresh, frozen, canned, or dried fruits and vegetables	Vegetables prepared in butter, cream, or other sauces
Breads and Cereals	Homemade baked goods using unsaturated oils sparingly, angel food cake, low-fat crackers, low-fat cookies	Commercial baked goods: pies, cakes, doughnuts, croissants, pastries, muffins, biscuits, high-fat crackers, high-fat cookies
	Rice, Pasta	Egg noodles
	Whole-grain breads and cereals (oatmeal, whole wheat, rye, bran, multigrain, etc.)	Breads in which eggs are major ingredient
Fats and Oils	Baking cocoa	Chocolate
	Unsaturated vegetable oils: corn, olive, rapeseed (canola oil), safflower, sesame, soybean, sunflower Margarine or shortening made from one of the unsaturated oils listed above	Butter, coconut oil, palm oil, palm kernel oil, lard, bacon fat
	Diet margarine	
	Mayonnaise, salad dressing made with unsaturated oils listed above	Dressings made with egg yolk
	Low-fat dressings	
	Seeds and nuts	Coconut

Source: National Cholesterol Education Program. (1989). *Report of the Expert Panel on Detection, Evaluation, and Treatment of High Blood Cholesterol in Adults.* U.S. Department of Health and Human Services, Public Health Service, National Institutes of Health. NIH publication No. 89–2925. p. 39.

4.   Replace whole milk with skim milk and nonfat dry milk.

5.   Skim milk cheeses should be substituted for whole milk cheeses.

6.   Tub margarines of safflower, sunflower, or corn oil are preferred over stick margarines made of the same oils. The reason is the stick margarines have a lower content of polyunsaturated oils.

7.   When you are eating out, avoid foods described in the following terms on the menu:

●   Buttery, buttered, or in butter sauce

●   Sauteed, fried, pan-fried, or crispy

●   Creamed, cream sauce, or "in its own gravy"

●   Au gratin, parmesan, in cheese sauce

●   Au lait, a la mode, or au fromage (with cheese)

●   Marinated, stewed, basted, or en casserol

●   Prime, hash, pot pie, hollandaise

Here is a sample menu that is low in total fat, saturated fat, and cholesterol:

Breakfast

1/2 grapefruit
1 ounce whole-grain cereal
1/2 cup skim milk
Black coffee

Lunch

1 cup navy bean soup

1 oat bran muffin, with polyunsaturated margarine
Lettuce and tomato salad with polyunsaturated oil/vinegar dressing
1 apple
1 cup skim milk

Dinner

3 oz baked chicken, skin removed
1 baked potato
1/2 cup broccoli
1 slice French bread
Polyunsaturated margarine
1/2 cup orange sherbet

Snacks

Graham/saltine crackers
Carrot sticks
Milk

Many researchers believe that dietary fiber that is water soluble—the type found in oat products, dried beans and peas, and many fruits and vegetables—helps lower blood cholesterol (Anderson, 1988). Since these foods are also very low in fat and contain no cholesterol, patients can be encouraged to include moderate amounts in a cholesterol-lowering diet.

A special type of fat, omega-3 fatty acids, is found in oily fish like salmon, mackerel, haddock, and other cold water fish. In populations who consume large quantities of fish, like the Greenland Eskimos, heart disease is virtually nonexistent. While the value of omega-3 fatty acids in preventing heart disease remains unclear, patients should be encouraged to eat fish often. Fish is still fairly low in fat and calories compared with other protein foods.

HIGH BLOOD PRESSURE

High blood pressure enhances deposits of cholesterol from the blood into the arterial wall, and thus it is a primary risk factor for developing atherosclerosis. There is no doubt that hypertension is a genetic disease. It is much more common in blacks than in whites. Blood pressure also rises with age. Formerly, it was believed that this rise was a normal part of aging. However, comparisons of other cultures, such as Eskimos in Greenland, African Bushmen, and others, showed no rise in blood pressure with age (Grundy, 1983). Japan and China have levels even higher than in the U.S.

The difference appears to lie in the diet, particularly in the levels of sodium in the diet. Another risk factor is overweight. This risk is independent of the amount of sodium in the diet.

The association of high blood pressure, or hypertension, with obesity has long been recognized (Eliahou, 1992). The Framingham study showed that an excess of body weight only 20 percent over ideal weight was associated with an eightfold increase in the incidence of high blood pressure later in life. Abdominal obesity is especially associated with high blood pressure.

The goal of treatment for hypertension is to achieve a blood pressure of 140/90mmHg or less while controlling other cardiovascular risk factors (National Institutes of Health, 1993). Lifestyle modifications, including weight loss, increased physical activity, and moderation of dietary sodium and alcohol intake, are the first line of treatment for mild, high blood pressure and should be tried for three to six months before starting drug therapy. Even with drug therapy, lifestyle modifications should continue.

Most importantly, obese individuals with high blood pressure should restrict calories and increase physical activity to lose weight. Weight loss of as little as 10 pounds will help lower blood pressure (National Institutes of Health, 1993).

Since excessive alcohol intake can raise blood pressure and make drug therapy less effective, alcohol intake should be limited. Alcohol is also a concentrated source of calories that supplies minimal vitamins or minerals. At a maximum, alcoholic beverages should be limited to one ounce of ethanol daily (two ounces of 100 proof whiskey, eight ounces of wine, or 24 ounces of beer).

Many studies show that blood pressure responds to reduced sodium intake, though the response of each individual varies. Blacks, older people, and individuals with high blood pressure seem to be more responsive to sodium intake. The National Institutes of Health (1993) recommends that individuals with mild, high blood pressure consume no more than 2.3 grams of sodium daily. Because dietary potassium, calcium, and magnesium intake may be related to blood pressure, adequate intake of these minerals is recommended.

Salt is by far the most plentiful source of sodium in American diets. The first step is to help the patient reduce the amount of salt in his diet (Connor, 1986). Helping to educate the patient about the amount of sodium in the diet and increasing his awareness of sodium in common foods will help him break the salt habit. This isn't accomplished overnight, and many people have acquired their taste for salt over many years. Therefore, it may take many months for them to unlearn the salt habit.

Sodium is an essential mineral that helps regulate water balance in the tissues. It comes from food and the salt that is added to foods. At least one-third of the sodium in American diets comes from the foods eaten. The rest is added via the salt shaker at the table and during cooking. Salt is a compound made of sodium and chloride, and roughly 40 percent of table salt is sodium. Salt is found in foods and even in products such as toothpaste.

Williams (1976) has offered some helpful hints for counseling your patients about using less salt in foods. It is difficult to adhere to lower levels of sodium at first. After several months this becomes easier. Here are a few suggestions for patients who are having difficulties with low-sodium diets:

- Stop adding salt at the table. Get rid of the shaker by putting it out of sight or throwing it away.

- If foods seem too bland without added salt, sprinkle them with fresh lemon juice instead. A number of companies are producing canned and frozen products with reduced amounts of sodium. Many varied spices can be substituted for salt, to produce a more tasty product. For example, try adding green pepper, mace, onion, paprika, and parsley to potatoes, or using bay leaf, dry mustard, green pepper, marjoram, fresh mushrooms, etc., with beef.

- Some vegetables are naturally high in sodium, such as artichokes, beet greens, carrots, celery, chard, kale, spinach, and whole hominy.

CANCER

Obesity appears to increase risk of developing certain types of cancer. In a study of the American Cancer Society (Garfinkle, 1985), cancer of the endometrium, uterus, cervix, ovary, gallbladder, and breast was increased in obese women. Prostate and colorectal cancer were increased in obese men.

The National Cancer Institute gives specific dietary recommendations to help prevent cancer (Butrum, 1988). These include:

- Reduce fat intake to 30 percent or less of total calories.
- Increase fiber intake to 20 to 30 grams daily.
- Include a variety of vegetables and fruits daily.
- Avoid obesity.
- Consume alcoholic beverages in moderation, if at all.
- Minimize consumption of salt-cured, salt-pickled, and smoked foods.

In addition to these recommendations, The National Cancer Institute recently launched a multimillion dollar campaign to encourage Americans to eat more fruits and vegetables. The campaign, called "Five a Day for Better Health," recommends eating at least five servings of fruits and vegetables daily. Fruits and vegetables are rich in dietary fiber and contain compounds called antioxidants which may help prevent certain cancers.

ELDERLY INDIVIDUALS

Elderly obese patients have special needs, due to the physiological, socioeconomic, and psychological changes that come with aging. Because there are so many differences among persons of the same age, and the effects of past nutrition and physical fitness can vary so widely, diets for elderly patients must be individualized, just as for younger persons.

Obesity is common in the over-60 population. About 18 percent of men and one-half of women are obese (Frankle, 1987). Older adults may have become obese from a simple factor such as not reducing intake of food as they became more sedentary, or more complicated reasons, as when medication increases appetite. As mentioned, nurses won't see many cases of gross obesity in elderly persons because most morbidly obese people die at a younger age.

Body composition changes occurring with age tend to make blood levels for drugs potentially higher in older persons than in their younger counterparts. Weight may decline, but the proportion of body fat increases, doubling in men and increasing by 50 percent in older women (Andres, 1985).

Drugs can also interfere with the absorption of ordinary nutrients. Many times complaints of chronic diarrhea which may be due to drug-induced malabsorption aren't followed up, and malnutrition results. Malabsorption of thiamine, folate, vitamin B12, fats, calcium, phosphate, and iron may lead to problems with osteoporosis, osteomalacia, and anemia, all of which may be mistakenly believed to be due to advanced age (Guthrie, 1988).

Elderly persons are also far more likely to self-prescribe and self-medicate than any other age group. Over-the-counter (OTC) drugs account for two of every five drugs taken by older persons. In addition, 80 percent of the elderly also use alcohol, prescribed drugs, or both (Posner, 1979). The most common OTC agents used by elderly persons include analgesics, cough and cold remedies (often alcohol-based), vitamins, external analgesics, laxatives, antihistamines, antidiarrheals, caffeine, nicotine, and antacids. It may be difficult to find out what products an older person is actually using, since he or she may not remember all the prescription and OTC products he takes. One good way to determine what an older person is taking is to ask the patient to bring in all medications, even the common drugstore medications not usually thought of as "drugs," and to evaluate their effects.

Instituting a special diet late in life can be difficult. Food habits, traditions, and food choices developed over a lifetime can't be easily erased, even for compelling health reasons. It is also not easy to accept

diet restrictions in the face of the other losses the elderly are often confronted with. Old age can be a terrible time of losses: friends, spouse, family, home, independence, and financial security. The loss of familiar and "comforting" foods can be disturbing because food is at least something that can be controlled.

Other factors may be involved, too. Consider an elderly man whose dentures don't fit right and cause him pain. If he can't afford to have his dentures fixed, he may resort to eating foods that can be consumed without teeth. If he can't afford to buy and prepare well-balanced diets and dietary supplements, he may resort to easily handled foods such as bread, mashed potatoes, and other easily swallowed, high-carbohydrate foods. Or think of an elderly woman who lives alone and whose arthritis is crippling. It may be nearly impossible for her to go to the supermarket to buy healthful and nutritious foods. She may also have trouble opening jars and preparing meats and fresh vegetables. Living alone and being alone may make her revert to easily prepared but nonnutritious foods. She may also have no particular desire to make meals, both because of her painful hands and because she may think, "What's the use, it's just me now."

These two elderly persons are very typical of the people the nurse will be working with. An understanding of the special nutrition needs of elderly individuals will make it much easier to design a diet for them, or to counsel them about the need to change part or all of their daily diet.

The best success usually can be obtained by an educational approach that stresses the importance of nutrition and explains the reduced calorie needs of the body. The patient should be encouraged to decrease food intake and increase activity levels, and eat more complex carbohydrates which are filling and low in fat and calories.

Calcium is also of special concern for elderly patients. In recent times, Americans have learned that an adequate intake of calcium is important to good health, particularly in postmenopausal women, and as a guard against osteoporosis or osteomalacia. The calcium needs of the elderly are at least equivalent to those of younger adults. Some people who have had long-term calcium deficiencies, either due to insufficient intake during adulthood or by an as-yet-undefined defect in adulthood, should have greater calcium intake. The seemingly obvious answer would be an increase in milk consumption. However, this is often too expensive and unpopular among the aged. When milk or milk products are contraindicated, older patients can take calcium gluconate or calcium lactate.

Phosphorus may be far more plentiful in the diet due to ingestion of large amounts of meat and soft drinks by some people. The higher intake of phosphorus may disrupt the calcium/phosphorus ratio, unless enough calcium is added to restore the balance.

Sodium restriction has become a familiar phrase to patients with congestive heart failure, hypertension, cirrhosis of the liver, and all other conditions where extracellular fluid retention is a problem. Controlling sodium levels may be a particularly difficult problem for mature and elderly adults whose physicians prescribe low-sodium diets, for two main reasons (Goodhart, 1980):

1. It is difficult for a patient to get meals that are low in sodium if he eats in restaurants or with other persons who aren't restricting sodium in their diets.

2. By lowering the palatability of diets, sodium restriction may lead to lowered consumption of food and thus to deficiencies of other essential nutrients.

Many health-care professionals have found that re-educating elderly persons about the importance of low-sodium (and, if necessary, substituting sodium-free condiments and flavorings) seems to help. In such cases, it is of paramount importance to motivate the older patient to control sodium intake.

In animals, restricting calories has long been linked to improved life span. Since caloric balance depends on intake versus energy expenditure, it is logical that as a person grows less active, fewer calories will be needed. Reducing calories alone isn't the goal, however. The true goal is to balance a healthful level of exercise with a nutritious diet.

Obese elderly individuals may need to make a special effort to eat a balanced, healthy diet. Programs such as the Home Delivered Meals program or the Meals On Wheels program can be a lifesaver for older individuals who are homebound. With Meals On Wheels, a hot, nutritious meal is delivered to the homes of elderly persons at least once a day, Monday through Friday.

Other programs such as the Congregate Meals program enable older persons to share one meal a day at least five days a week with their peers. Free transportation is often provided.

CHILDREN AND ADOLESCENTS

Just as adult obesity is increasing in prevalence, so is pediatric obesity. About one in four children are overweight, and the numbers are on the rise. Overweight children often, though not always, grow up to be overweight adults. The older the child is at onset of obesity and the more severe the obesity, the greater the chance the child will remain obese as an adult (Dietz, 1992).

Childhood obesity can have severe psychosocial implications. Children who are overweight should not be put on weight loss diets. Many obese children eat the same or fewer calories than normal-weight children (Dietz, 1992). Rather, healthy eating and exercise behaviors should be encouraged to slow the rate of weight gain and to allow height to catch up with weight. Severely restricting calories in childhood could interfere with normal growth or promote the development of eating disorders (Johnston, 1985).

Diet counseling of young children should focus on the parents' role as "gatekeepers" of foods brought into the house. If diet assessment reveals the child is eating too many calorie-dense foods such as potato chips, cookies, soft drinks, candy or ice cream, the parents should be encouraged to limit (not necessarily omit) purchase of these foods and try to emphasize healthy meals and snacks.

When counseling older children and adolescents, focusing too much on the parental role may be counterproductive if the child is striving to achieve autonomy. Diet counselors should also be sure that an adolescent who wishes to lose weight really needs to. At any given time, 75 to 95 percent of adolescents girls are dissatisfied with their weight (Obesity Update, 1993).

The nurse should encourage the entire family to adopt healthy eating habits for the benefit of both the patient and other family members. This also avoids singling out the obese child as different or the reason certain foods cannot be kept in the house.

If the child isn't active enough, which is often the case, parents need to encourage activity. This might mean limiting television viewing, allowing adequate time for safe, outdoor play, joining a sports team, or planning family activities of nature hikes, swimming, volleyball, sliding, or skiing. Although an activity might not be strenuous enough to be considered aerobic, any extra activity helps burn calories.

As with adult obesity, prevention is more effective than treatment. Any child who is above the seventy-fifth percentile of weight for height should be monitored closely for development of obesity (The American Dietetic Association, 1989). Children and their parents should be encouraged to adopt healthy eating and exercise behaviors at an early age to help prevent obesity.

The next chapter examines one of the most crucial and often overlooked parts of any weight loss or weight maintenance program, exercise.

EXAM QUESTIONS

Chapter 9

Questions 75-83

75. Weighing 20 percent over ideal weight increases incidence of high blood pressure later in life:

    a. twofold
    b. fourfold
    c. sixfold
    d. eightfold

76. A desirable blood cholesterol level for adults is:

    a. less than 180mg/dl
    b. less than 200mg/dl
    c. 200-239mg/di
    d. less than 240mg/dl

77. Which type of cholesterol increases risk of coronary heart disease the most?

    a. very low-density lipoprotein cholesterol
    b. low-density lipoprotein cholesterol
    c. intermediate-density lipoprotein cholesterol
    d. high-density lipoprotein cholesterol

78. Which of the following is recommended to help reduce the risk of developing cancer?

    a. eat adequate amounts of protein
    b. reduce exposure to food additives
    c. eat 6 to 8 servings of breads daily
    d. increase fiber intake 20 to 30 grams daily

79. The main dietary goal for obese individuals with type II diabetes is:

    a. to cut down on the total number of calories
    b. to cut down on calories from simple carbohydrates
    c. to increase the glycemic index of foods
    d. to decrease fat intake

80. For an individual with a blood cholesterol level of 260mg/dl, what therapy should be tried first?

    a. drug therapy
    b. Step-One diet and exercise
    c. Step-Two diet and exercise
    d. no intervention is necessary for this cholesterol level

81. The American Diabetes Association recommends what level of fiber intake daily?

    a. up to 10 grams daily
    b. up to 25 grams daily
    c. up to 40 grams daily
    d. up to 55 grams daily

82. Which of the following foods may lower blood cholesterol levels?

    a. omega-3 fatty acids
    b. saturated fats
    c. insoluble fiber
    d. soluble fiber

83. Treatment for obese children should be designed to:

    a. slow the rate of weight gain
    b. allow for a weekly weight loss of one pound
    c. limit weekly weight losses to 1/2 pound
    d. obese children should not be treated

CHAPTER 10

EXERCISE INTERVENTION
A CRITICAL INGREDIENT

CHAPTER OBJECTIVE

After studying this chapter, you will be able to describe the benefits of regular exercise and specify guidelines for exercising safely.

LEARNING OBJECTIVES

After studying this chapter, you will be able to:

1. Identify parts of an exercise prescription.

2. Discuss appropriate type, intensity, duration, frequency, and progression of exercise for obese patients.

3. Recognize behaviors that help patients continue exercising regularly.

4. Describe specific exercises for the severely obese person.

INTRODUCTION

Exercise may well be the only ingredient missing from a successful lifetime weight control program. Adding a 45-minute walk three days per week would produce a yearly weight loss of nine pounds for a person weighing 160 pounds (Walberg-Rankin, 1992). Combining exercise with dietary restriction can speed up weight loss, help tone muscles, and reduce risk for chronic disease. This chapter will look at the benefits of exercise, then discuss some specific types of exercises.

BENEFITS OF EXERCISE

Physical activity has long been known to be beneficial for optimal health. Exercise maintains good muscle tone, stimulates the circulation, and is also an aid to digestion. Exercise is also a stress-reliever. Strenuous exercise helps relax muscle tension, and has a tranquilizing effect, probably partially due to the release of endorphins.

In a study of 10,269 men who graduated from Harvard College, Paffenbarger and colleagues (1993) found that moderately vigorous exercise was associated with lower overall death rates and lower death rates from coronary heart disease. In this study, an exercise program reduced death risk 23 percent.

In a similar 16-year follow-up of Norwegian men, Sandvik and colleagues (1993) also found that greater levels of physical fitness are associated with lower risk of death from cardiovascular disease and death from all causes.

The good news is that people don't have to exercise at a high intensity to achieve lower levels of cardio-vascular risk. In a study of 102 sedentary adult women (Duncan, 1991), women were randomly as-signed to walking 4.8 kilometers daily for five days at an aerobic pace, at a brisk walk, or at a leisurely stroll. Although the aerobic walking group achieved better cardiorespiratory fitness, all groups had equally favorable changes in cardiovascular risk profile.

Regular physical activity:
- Reduces blood pressure,
- Lowers levels of dangerous low-density lipopro-tein (LDL) cholesterol levels,
- Raises levels of protective high-density lipopro-tein (HDL) cholesterol levels,
- Helps stabilize blood sugar,
- Burns calories and aids in weight loss,
- Relieves stress,
- Tones muscles,
- Helps people look and feel their best.

How does exercise help promote weight loss and weight control? When diet and exercise are com-bined, regular exercise increases the rate of weight loss. In addition, an obese person will burn more calories than his lean counterpart when doing the same tasks. Although cutting calories has the most dramatic effect on weight loss, regular exercise can also make an important contribution. Exercise by it-self can help a person lose weight by increasing the expenditure of energy. One doesn't need to cut back the number of calories so strictly. For example, if one decides to cut back 500 calories a day, or 3,500

calories a week (the amount needed to lose one pound), by adding an activity that burns 250 calories per day, one can cut merely 250 calories instead of 500 from the diet and still trim 500 calories a day. Table 10.1 lists the approximate energy cost of many different activities. As shown in the table, the more a person weighs, the greater the energy cost of the activity.

Another benefit of regular exercise is a cosmetic one. Regular exercise is the only way to reduce the "flab factor." Without combining exercise with diet, the body will be flabby no matter how much weight is lost. As Dr. Simonson (1983) has written, no diet plan ever devised, no matter what anyone says, will prevent sags and bags if one loses more than 10 or 20 pounds and is over 35 or 40 years of age.

The only antidote to the flab factor is regular exer-cise, which will tone the muscles and give the skin a tighter appearance. This will ultimately make a per-son look trimmer because muscle tissue takes up less volume than fatty tissue. High-protein diets are especially prone to cause flab, because along with losing fat tissue one will be losing muscle tissue, or the tissue that helps give the body its shape. The result will be a saggy, baggy, although thinner, body. Regular exercise preserves lean body mass,and helps a greater portion of the weight loss to be from fat rather than muscle tissue.

Individuals who are inactive have relatively low en-ergy needs, and if they wish to reach an ideal body weight, they must rigidly control food intake. Dr. Jean Mayer (Stein, 1986) has said, to avoid obesity, one must either exercise more or feel hungry all of one's life.

Far from making one feel exhausted, vigorous exer-cise delivers a sense of energy and vitality. As one continues to exercise, muscle tissue replaces fat tis-sue, and muscle tissue requires more calories to maintain than fatty tissue does.

Table 10.1 Energy Expenditure by Body Weight in Selected Physical Activities

Activity	Calories per min per lb body weight	Body weight (lb)			
		150	200	250	300
Archery	.030	4.5	6.0	7.5	9.0
Basketball	.063	9.5	12.6	15.8	18.9
Bicycling					
(5.5 mph)	.029	4.4	5.8	7.3	8.7
(9.4 mph)	.045	6.8	9.0	11.3	13.5
Canoeing (leisure)	.020	3.0	4.0	5.0	6.0
Chopping wood	.039	5.9	7.8	9.8	11.7
Cleaning house	.027	4.1	5.4	6.8	8.1
Climbing hills	.055	8.3	11.0	13.8	16.5
Cooking	.021	3.2	4.2	5.3	6.3
Dancing (slow)	.023	3.5	4.6	5.8	6.9
Dancing (fast)	.046	6.9	9.2	11.5	13.8
Digging (trenches)	.066	9.9	13.2	16.5	19.8
Field hockey	.061	9.2	12.2	15.3	18.3
Fishing	.028	4.2	5.6	7.0	8.4
Food shopping	.027	4.1	5.4	6.8	8.1
Football	.060	9.0	12.0	15.0	18.0
Golf	.039	5.9	7.8	9.8	11.7
Horse riding (trot)	.050	7.5	10.0	12.5	15.0
Ironing	.022	3.3	4.4	5.5	6.6
Lying at ease	.010	1.5	2.0	2.5	3.0
Mopping floor	.027	4.1	5.4	6.8	8.1
Mowing	.051	7.7	10.2	12.8	15.3
Painting (house)	.035	5.3	7.0	8.8	10.5
Racquetball	.096	14.4	19.2	24.0	28.8
Raking	.025	3.8	5.0	6.3	7.5
Running					
9 min/mile	.088	13.2	17.6	22.0	26.4
12 min/mile	.061	9.2	12.2	15.3	18.3
Sawing by hand	.034	5.1	6.8	8.5	10.2
Scrubbing floors	.050	7.5	10.0	12.5	15.0
Sewing	.011	1.7	2.2	2.8	3.3
Sitting	.010	1.5	2.0	2.5	3.0
Skiing (downhill)	.050	7.5	10.0	12.5	15.0
Standing quietly	.012	1.8	2.4	3.0	3.6
Swimming					
Backstroke	.077	11.5	15.4	19.3	23.1
Breast stroke	.074	11.1	14.8	18.5	22.2
Crawl (fast)	.071	10.7	14.2	17.8	21.3
Crawl (slow)	.058	8.7	11.6	14.5	17.4
Table tennis	.031	4.7	6.2	7.8	9.3
Tennis	.050	7.5	10.0	12.5	15.0
Typing	.012	1.8	2.4	3.0	3.6
Volleyball	.023	3.5	4.6	5.8	6.9
Walking					
3 mph	.031	4.7	6.2	7.8	9.3
4 mph	.041	6.2	8.2	10.3	12.3
Wallpapering	.022	3.3	4.4	5.5	6.6
Weeding	.033	5.0	6.6	8.3	9.9
Window cleaning	.027	4.1	5.4	6.8	8.1

Source: Perri, M.G., Nezu, A.M., Viegener, B.J. (1992). *Improving the Long-Term Management of Obesity.* New York: John Wiley & Sons, 188–189.

Some individuals are concerned that exercise will increase appetite. On the contrary, regular exercise usually decreases appetite. Dr. Jean Mayer's group (Stein, 1986) showed that food intake declines as movement is made from low- to moderate-activity occupations. Exercise also helps prevent the decline in metabolic rate that sometimes occurs with prolonged dieting.

EXERCISING SAFELY

According to guidelines of the American College of Sports Medicine (1991), healthy men 40 years of age and younger and healthy women 50 years of age and younger do not need to consult a doctor before beginning a sensible and gradual exercise program. Older healthy individuals do not need to consult a doctor if they begin an exercise program of moderate intensity (exercise that can be comfortably continued for up to an hour at the individual's current level of fitness) and progress slowly.

The American College of Sports Medicine recommends that a doctor be consulted before beginning an exercise program if:

1. The patient is older than 40 years for men and 50 years for women and is beginning a vigorous exercise program (a challenging regimen that tires out the individual within 20 minutes at current level of fitness).

2. The patient has two or more risk factors for heart disease (such as high blood pressure, high blood cholesterol levels, cigarette smoking, diabetes mellitus, family history of atherosclerotic disease in parents or siblings prior to age 55).

3. The patient has symptoms of heart disease (such pain or pressure in the left midchest area, neck, shoulder, or arm during or right after exercise; shortness of breath; faintness or dizziness; palpitations, or claudication).

4. The patient has known heart disease or other diseases that might require special attention, such as pulmonary disease, diabetes, or bone or joint problems.

These are general guidelines; discretion should be used for each patient individually.

Patients should always be advised to start an exercise program slowly and build up gradually. Walking is a good way to start. All that is needed is a good pair of walking shoes. Patients can walk at their own pace for a comfortable distance. If pain occurs during exercise, the patient should slow down or stop. A sensible, gradual exercise program should be painless.

Preparing for exercise. It's important to prepare for exercise by allowing time for stretching, a warm-up period, activity period, then a cool-down period. Stretching is important because it increases flexibility and helps prepare the body for exercise. Stretching should be done every time the patient exercises, just before warming up. Stretching should also be done after exercise to cool down. The following are some suggested stretches for various parts of the body:

Neck. Stand or sit in a chair, with your arms relaxed at the sides, looking ahead. Now, slowly tilt the head to the shoulder on a slow count of 4, returning to your original position on 4 more counts. Stretch 4 times.

Sides. Stand with legs comfortably apart, toes pointing straight ahead, knees relaxed, and both arms stretched overhead. Then stretch slowly to one side on a count of 8; hold this position for a count of 10; then slowly return to the original position on a count of 8. Do this 4 times. Then stretch slowly to the other side and repeat.

Shoulders. Stand with legs comfortably apart, knees relaxed, holding a towel in your right hand. Drop the right hand over the right shoulder to the upper back. Bring the left hand under the left shoulder toward the upper back, grabbing the towel. Pull the towel slowly with the left hand. When a stretch in the shoulders is felt, hold this position for a count of 10, or about 10 seconds. Then pull the towel with the right hand, until a stretch in the shoulder is felt, Hold this position for a count of 10. Reverse the position of hands, and repeat. Do this 4 times. With practice the patient will be able to do the stretch without the towel.

Calf and Achilles tendon stretch. Stand a little more than an arm's length in front of a wall, with heels flat on the floor or ground. Place hands, at shoulder height, firmly against the wall, then slowly lean forward with legs and back straight. Try to touch shoulders and chest to the wall, turning the face to the side. When a pull in your calves is felt, hold the position for a count of 20, or about 20 seconds, keeping the heels flat on the floor. Return to the first position. Repeat this stretch 4 times.

Lower back and hamstring stretch. While seated on the floor with legs outstretched and feet together, press the backs of the legs against the floor. Slowly bend forward from the hips, keeping the back straight. Reach toward the toes and touch them if possible. Or, if the patient can't reach his feet, grasp the ankles. When the tension in the back of the legs is felt, hold the position for 10 seconds, then return to the original position. Do this stretch 4 times.

Once the patient has stretched, a warm-up period comes next. About five minutes of warming-up helps get muscles, joints, and the cardiovascular system going. For example, five minutes of easy walking helps get the body ready for further activity. A cooling-down period is important, to allow the body

to return to the level it was at before exercise began. The best way to cool-down is to continue the activity at an easy pace for 5 to 10 more minutes. If walking at a brisk pace, slow down a little, swing the arms less vigorously, and take shorter steps. If swimming, slow the strokes until breathing returns to normal.

THE EXERCISE PRESCRIPTION

Begin a discussion by having the patient estimate how much exercise he or she currently does. Discuss any regular exercise or activity plus day-to-day activities such as walking to work or using the stairs instead of the elevator. The health practitioner and patient can then jointly develop an exercise prescription. A trained exercise physiologist can assist in evaluating high risk patients and developing an exercise prescription.

According to the American College of Sports Medicine (1991), an exercise prescription is a recommended regimen of physical activity designed to enhance fitness, promote health, and ensure safety. An exercise prescription has five main elements that must be addressed:

1. Type of exercise,
2. Intensity of exercise,
3. Duration of exercise,
4. Frequency of exercise, usually described on a weekly basis, and
5. Progression to more intense and longer exercise sessions.

TYPE OF EXERCISE

Any regular, rhythmic exercise that continually works the large muscles of the body is considered aerobic exercise. Examples of vigorous aerobic activity that conditions the heart and lungs if done for at least 15 to 30 minutes include:

- cross-country skiing
- ice hockey
- jogging
- jumping rope
- rowing
- running in place
- stationary biking

Some activities that condition the heart and lungs if done briskly include:

- bicycling
- basketball
- calisthenics
- racquetball
- swimming
- tennis (singles)
- walking

Activities that can be fun, help you to get moving, and use up calories but do not usually condition the heart and lungs include:

- baseball
- bowling
- football
- golf
- volleyball

Walking. Walking is enjoying a new surge of popularity largely because people of any age can walk, and it requires nothing more than a good pair of walking shoes. It uses all the major muscles of the body, can be done at varying levels, from a brisk walk to race walking, can provide just as many benefits as jogging, and produces much less strain on the knees and ankles than jogging does. Walking has also become a social event in some areas. In many larger cities, groups gather to walk through historic sections of the city or to special sites.

Nearly every program starts with a gentle pace of walking for a prescribed time or distance. For the extremely overweight person, it may be best to think in terms of blocks instead of miles. Soon it is easy to work up to a half-hour of walking, then an hour. A good measure of the speed to aim for is a walk brisk enough that the patient is breathing heavily but can still talk. Even if the patient starts out slowly, he should work up to a pace of about 4 miles per hour. Walking as little as 15 minutes a day can lead to a weight loss of up to 26 pounds a year.

Swimming. Swimming, another good exercise that can be done year-round, also helps increase the heart rate and moves all major muscles. This is often an excellent exercise for older persons because it avoids strain on the joints of the lower leg and arms. However, to be effective, swimming must be continuous and vigorous, beginning slowly at first but working up to about a half-hour. One hour of swimming will use up about 670 calories, so that every five hours of swimming equals the loss of one pound.

Cycling. Cycling is excellent for the heart, lower body muscles, and for weight loss. One can cycle nearly everywhere on the streets and side roads, or on a stationary bike in bad weather. Thirty minutes of vigorous cycling, or a speed of about 9 mph, will burn about 210 calories.

Stair-climbing. Stair-climbing is very demanding physically, and may not be good for persons who are moderately or greatly overweight. To stair-climb, a person walks up and down a flight of stairs, working up to a half hour. Climbing should be done steadily and rhythmically, resting between flights if necessary. Apparently stair-climbing uses so much energy that just climbing an extra two flights of stairs a day can lead to a weight loss of 10 to 12 pounds a year.

Stepping. This is an exercise that is well suited to persons who like to exercise in private, but it is fairly strenuous. All that is needed is a step or stool about 7 inches high. One steps up on the stool with one foot, then brings the other foot up, then steps back down with one foot, then brings the other foot down. This is a fairly strenuous exercise because stepping means lifting the total weight of the body up. It's best to start out with only four or five step-ups, then build up. Also, very heavy persons or those that are out of condition should wait until less strenuous exercises have been mastered. Working up from four or five steps to a half hour without stress is the goal.

Jogging. In many programs, jogging has been replaced with walking or alternated with walking for best results. Jogging may be too strenuous for some overweight persons; it also can lead to injuries and, of course, to dropping out of the exercise program. For others, it provides great aerobic benefits.

INTENSITY OF EXERCISE

All activity is of benefit, but to condition the heart and lungs, the activity must be brisk enough to raise heart rate and breathing. No matter which exercise you choose, it is important to start slowly and build up gradually.

A general guideline is that the activity should make you breath a little harder, but not so hard that you cannot talk to someone. Closer guidelines are based on heart rate. The harder the body works, the faster the heart will beat. The goal is to get the heart beating in a medium zone, neither too quickly nor too slowly.

Maximum heart rate is the upper rate limit characteristic of an age group. This is generally estimated by taking 220 and subtracting a person's age. Sustained, maximum heart contraction is dangerous. Therefore, the target heart rate for exercising is 60 to 75 percent of maximum heart rate (see Table 10.2). A beginner should aim for the lower number of the target zone, whereas someone who has been exercising regularly should aim for the higher number in the range.

To find your pulse while exercising, place the tips of the thumb and first two fingers on either side of the throat, just below the jawbone. Here the carotid artery can be easily felt. Then, using a watch with a second hand, count the number of pulsations felt in six seconds and add a zero to that number. Another good pulse spot is at the wrist. Press gently with the index and middle fingers on the thumb side of the wrist; don't use the thumb to count the pulsations because it has a pulse of its own.

DURATION OF EXERCISE

To condition the heart and lungs, the heart must beat within the target zone for 15 to 30 continuous minutes during the active phase of exercise. For the person who isn't used to exercise, however, a few minutes in the lower end of the target heart range is a good place to start. The exercise session should always be preceded with at least a five minute warm-up period and followed by a five minute cool-down period:

Exercise Session

Warm-up	5 minutes
Exercise	15 to 30 minutes
Cool down	5 minutes
Total Time	25 to 40 minutes

Table 10.2 Target Heart Rates

Age in years	Target Zone (beats per minute) (60-75% of maximum)	Average Maximum Heart Rate 100% (beats per minute)
20	120–150	200
25	117–146	195
30	114–142	190
35	111–138	185
40	108–135	180
45	105–131	175
50	102–127	170
55	99–123	165
60	96–120	160
65	93–116	155
70	90–113	150

Source: National Institutes of Health Fact Sheet on Exercise.

FREQUENCY OF EXERCISE

It is not necessary to exercise every day to reap the benefits of exercise. Exercise physiologists advise exercise three to five times weekly. Even people who only exercise three times weekly will be amazed at how much better they'll feel. Regular exercise three to five times weekly will firm up muscles, increase energy level, burn off extra calories, and reduce stress and tension.

PROGRESSION

With any new exercise routine, a person should start slowly and build up gradually. As a person continues to exercise, the exercise becomes easier and intensity and duration of the exercise session can be gradually increased.

How fast to progress with more vigorous and longer exercise sessions depends on many factors, such as a person's age, health status, preferences, and goals. Most people can gradually progress to a regular exercise routine of appropriate duration and intensity over six to eight weeks. Very overweight individuals and individuals who have not exercised in a long time may progress more slowly. Individuals who are in better physical condition to start with may progress more quickly. If the patient experiences stiffness or soreness after exercise, he or she is progressing too fast.

STICKING WITH IT

Just as dieting is never easy, getting into and staying with an exercise program isn't always easy. However, there are some ways the nurse can help the patient stick with it and eventually lead a more active life. The trick is to make activity a regular part of life, not merely a short-term effort.

Encourage them to try to think of ways to be more active at work, at home, and in other settings. Some examples include parking further away from a store so that one will have to walk a longer distance. Other measures, like reducing television time and substituting other activities, may help get some "couch potatoes" up and out of the deadly easy chair in front of the TV.

Another good idea is to search out local swimming pools and gymnasiums and the local YMCA and YWCA. Use facilities that are conveniently located near home or work.

Having good companionship during exercise can also be a great help, and in fact may be the key to keeping a patient active. For some persons, participating in a group activity, such as aerobics class, is the strongest factor that compels them to keep exercising. Finding a good walking companion or a group can help turn an ordinary brisk walk into an adventure. Social support is extremely important.

Finally, the activity has to be enjoyable or it stands a good chance of being dropped. Once a person becomes proficient in an activity and finds that he enjoys it, for companionship or better health, it is likely that it will become a permanent addition to a healthier life.

EXERCISES FOR SEVERELY OBESE PERSONS

For the person who is extremely overweight, it may be nearly impossible to jump right into a typi-cal exercise program (Foss, 1984). A more cautious approach, starting with a thorough checkup, is best. At Johns Hopkins Hospital, obese patients start with a sitting exercise program in which patients do exercises in a chair with no arms, then add a 5-minute walk every day. These patients are warned against participating in exercises such as jogging, rope jumping, weight-lifting, climbing stairs, one-legged exercises, or competitive sports, all of which can be dangerous to their health. Patients begin with three months or more of sitting exercises and walking, then advance to swimming, walking, or exercises on a stationary bicycle.

Some examples of beginning sitting exercises might include the following:

Seated jumping jacks. Swing arms overhead, touching the backs of the hands to each other, simultaneously moving the feet as far apart as possible. Return to starting position. Start with three repetitions, and work up to 10.

Side-stretchers. Raise left hand overhead with palm toward the ceiling. Place right hand on the hip or the arm of the chair, and lean to the right as far as possible. Stretch out four times. Now reverse the procedure, raising the right hand and placing the left hand on the hip, leaning to the left and stretching.

This gentle and gradual approach to exercise helps very overweight persons stick with it. As they cut down on their calories, good results are seen.

Chapter 11 examines ways nurses can help patients keep weight off permanently and avoid relapse.

EXAM QUESTIONS

Chapter 10

Questions 84-92

84. In a study of women walking 4.8 kilometers for exercise daily, which walking speed improved cardiovascular risk profile the most?

    a. aerobic pace
    b. brisk walk
    c. leisurely stroll
    d. all speeds improved cardiovascular risk profile

85. For a person weighing 160 pounds, adding a 45-minute walk, three days weekly would produce a yearly weight loss of about:

    a. 2 pounds
    b. 9 pounds
    c. 18 pounds
    d. 26 pounds

86. Regular physical activity:

    a. raises levels of high-density lipoprotein cholesterol
    b. raises blood glucose levels
    c. increases appetite
    d. depresses endorphins

87. The target heart rate for optimal conditioning of the heart and lungs during exercise is what percentage of maximum heart rate?

    a. 80-90%
    b. 60-75%
    c. 50-65%
    d. 35-45%

88. Which of the following is not an element of the exercise prescription?

    a. intensity of exercise
    b. progression of exercise
    c. duration of exercise
    d. cycle of exercise

89. Maximum heart rate is generally estimated by:

    a. multiplying pulse by 2.5
    b. multiplying target heart rate by 1.5
    c. taking 220 and adding a person's age
    d. taking 220 and subtracting a person's age

90. All of the following activities condition the heart and lungs except:

    a. baseball
    b. cross-country skiing
    c. stationary biking
    d. rowing

91. Which of the following individuals should consult a doctor before beginning a moderate exercise program?

    a. a healthy 60-year old women
    b. a 45 year-old women who smokes cigarettes
    c. a healthy 50-year old man
    d. a 35-year old man with high blood pressure and high blood cholesterol levels

92. Exercise physiologists recommend exercising how many days weekly?

    a. 2
    b. 3 to 5
    c. 6
    d. every day

CHAPTER 11

EVALUATION WEIGHT MAINTENANCE AND RELAPSE PREVENTION

CHAPTER OBJECTIVE

After reading this chapter, you will be able to identify factors that help patients achieve life-long dietary and exercise changes.

LEARNING OBJECTIVES

After studying this chapter, you will be able to:

1. Specify components of a comprehensive program that increase the likelihood of maintaining weight loss for the long-term.

2. Discuss key strategies to prevent relapse.

INTRODUCTION

Losing weight takes work, but weight loss is only the first step in lifetime weight control. The second, and perhaps more difficult step, is keeping the weight off. This chapter discusses continuous professional contact, social and peer support, exercise, and training in relapse prevention as measures to improve the likelihood of weight maintenance. Obesity is viewed as a chronic condition requiring long-term treatment.

A CONTINUOUS CARE MODEL

Few studies evaluate maintenance of weight loss over the long-term. Of those that do, results show that most individuals regain much of the weight lost (Perri, 1992). Physiological processes such as lowered metabolic rate and altered body chemistry can work against efforts to maintain weight loss. Feeling continually restricted and following a rigid diet over the long-term can also increase the likelihood of relapse.

Because of the strong possibility of relapse after weight loss, Dr. Michael Perri, a psychologist at the University of Florida in Gainesville, proposes a continuous care model for obesity management. The model asserts that obesity is a chronic condition that requires long-term care. After initial treatment for obesity, Perri (1993) advocates comprehensive programs that combine continuous professional contact, skills training in relapse prevention, social support, and exercise to enhance long-term weight maintenance.

ELEMENTS OF A SUCCESSFUL WEIGHT MAINTENANCE PROGRAM

Realistic Goals

The first step of setting realistic weight maintenance goals is to set realistic weight loss goals. If the nurse has helped the patient set realistic goals for weight loss, then maintaining those goals over the long-term will be easier. If a woman who is 5' 4" tall and weighs 200 pounds at the beginning of treatment set a goal weight of 120 pounds, maintenance of that weight would be extremely difficult, physiologically and psychologically. If her initial goal weight was to lose 20 pounds, or 10 percent of body weight, maintenance her reduced weight over the long-term would be easier.

Patients should not expect perfection in weight maintenance or complete adherence to a dietary or exercise program. Everyone's weight fluctuates and everyone occasionally indulges in high-calorie foods or gets off their exercise routine at some point. Individuals who have lost weight should expect that these things will happen and plan in advance how to handle them. The important thing is not to let such events derail the entire weight maintenance effort, but to get right back on track again.

Grilo and Brownell (1993) state that successful goals for weight maintenance are:

1. Specific (e.g., begin a walking program on "Tuesday morning before work," rather than "begin a walking program sometime next week");

2. Broken down into short- and long-term goals (e.g. walking 5 minutes longer each day toward an eventual goal of walking 45 minutes four times weekly); and

3. Require constant evaluation, looking at progress and problems.

Grilo and Brownell suggest that a person trying to maintain weight loss should keep sight of its many benefits, such as improved health, a higher level of fitness, more confidence, greater well-being, and feeling and looking better.

A Life-long Eating Plan

Adherance to a very restricted and rigid diet over the long-term is difficult and almost impossible for some people. Following a balanced diet that is low in fat and high in carbohydrate during the weight loss phase teaches diet principles that promote long-term weight maintenance.

Diets that are low in fat and high in complex carbohydrate and fiber offer a greater volume of food at a lower calorie level. The low-fat, high carbohydrate diet provides a greater degree of satiety and feeling of fullness, and helps to prevent overeating (Anderson, 1987). When an individual follows such a diet, an occasional high-fat or calorie-laden food will not have much impact on weight.

Continuous Professional Contact

Some professionals have tried providing "booster" sessions after weight loss to review and reinforce diet and exercise concepts learned during the weight loss phase. There are often three to six sessions held one to three months apart. After reviewing the literature, Perri (1992) concluded that such sessions are not as effective as they could be. Sessions may have been too far apart, with too little professional contact.

To be most effective, Perri states that professional contact must be frequent and geared specifically toward weight maintenance. Weight maintenance brings a whole new set of challenges as compared to weight loss. Therefore, therapist contact should focus on helping the patient anticipate high-risk situations, solve problems, and develop coping skills to prevent relapse. As an alternative to conventional appointments, Perri suggests having the patient telephone the therapist and mail in written activity and eating records.

Perri compared the weight maintenance of six groups to determine the impact of intensive and continuous professional contact. The first three groups had no continuous professional contact but the first group received only diet instruction; the second group received diet instruction plus behavior modification instruction; and the third group received diet and behavior modification instruction plus training in relapse prevention. The next three groups had the same initial treatment as each of the above three groups except that professional contact for six months after weight loss was added to their program.

The groups that had training in all three areas—diet, behavior modification, and relapse prevention—plus the continuous professional contact had the best weight maintenance of all groups and maintained most of their initial weight loss at both the six-month and twelve-month follow-up.

Social Support

Perri (1992) also compared the effects of long-term contact with a therapist or a peer support group on weight maintenance. Subjects in the peer support groups met bi-weekly. Other subjects had contact with their therapist on a bi-weekly basis. At 18 months after weight loss, both methods improved maintenance of weight loss as compared to conven-

tional behavior therapy with no continuous peer or professional contact.

Close family and friends of the patient can also help, or hinder, the patient's weight maintenance efforts. From the beginning, it's important for the patient to have the support of those around him. Without the support of family members or significant others, eating can be easily sabotaged. Here are some ways to enlist cooperation:

- Invite the patient's spouse to a counseling session, especially if he or she does most of the shopping for and preparation of foods.

- Ask for the family members' support, explain the gradual but lasting changes that can be made in the patient's diet, and keep them informed of the patient's progress.

- Ask family to help the patient cut down his or her exposure to the wrong types of foods, for example, not keeping these foods around, or, if they must have them, by keeping them out of sight.

- Work with a family member if he or she has similar dietary needs.

- If there are children at home, ask them to help with selection and preparation of foods.

- For anyone who lives alone, particularly older persons, have them ask friends for encouragement and support.

Help the patient prepare for possible problems with the people he lives with, and remind him to ask for, not demand, their help.

Regular Exercise

Just as exercise may well be the only ingredient missing from a weight loss program, it may also be the missing ingredient for successful weight maintenance. In fact, continuing exercise is one of the best predictors of successful weight maintenance.

In one study, only those subjects who continued exercising regularly maintained most of their weight loss after two years (Van Dale, 1990). In Perri's studies (1992), subjects in a weight maintenance program who had continuous therapist contact, behavioral training, social support, and 180 minutes of aerobic exercise weekly maintained 99 percent of their initial weight loss at the 18-month follow-up.

While following a rigid diet day after day requires constant vigilance, walking 30 minutes three to four times weekly is a much easier and more controllable activity for most people. Without making any conscientious changes in diet, walking one mile every day would help most individuals lose about 14 pounds a year.

Skills for Preventing Relapse

In the weight maintenance phase, the therapist must help the patient identify and cope with barriers to weight maintenance. The problems the patient encounters in the weight maintenance phase are different from those in the weight loss phase. The therapist and the patient must problem solve together and prevent minor slips from becoming major relapses.

In the relapse cycle, an individual confronts some type of high-risk situation which challenges eating control. The situation could be a social event, an argument with a spouse, or a stressful day. With no coping skills, the individual can lose control over his or her eating. This loss of control undermines the individual's confidence and self-esteem. Thoughts like "I really blew it this time, so I might as well wait until next week to get back on track" or "I'll never be able to keep my weight off" become self-fulfilling. One lapse leads to another, and soon the patient abandons all control, falls into total relapse, and regains much of the initial weight loss.

Perri (1992) and Brownell (1992) outline several strategies to help prevent relapse. First, the therapist should help the patient identify high-risk situations that could lead to loss of control over eating. The therapist might ask the patient to keep a record of high-risk situations over a few week's time, to list situations that have triggered loss of control in the past, or to imagine a high-risk situation.

Next, the therapist must help the patient develop skills for coping with his high-risk situations. This might mean bringing a low-calorie dish to a social gathering, planning ahead what to order at a restaurant, being assertive with friends or family, keeping certain foods out of the house, making a list of alternative activities when the urge to binge strikes, or even pre-planning a splurge. Patients may also want to have a plan of action in place if a certain amount of weight is re-gained.

The therapist should encourage the patient to practice and evaluate coping strategies. Oftentimes maintenance groups go out to a restaurant together or schedule a pot-luck meal to review coping strategies. Practicing these strategies builds self-confidence and gives the individual a feeling of control. Finally, the therapist must help the patient counter negative thoughts when he or she loses control.

LIFETIME WEIGHT CONTROL

Losing weight and keeping it off isn't easy. As seen in this course, there are physiological, socioeconomic, emotional, and behavioral reasons why we gain weight, and why the majority of us never take the excess pounds off. Overweight is one of America's greatest health problems. It is the major contributor to atherosclerotic disease and, in turn, to heart disease and stroke. Our mechanized society and the advent of television and leisure life have taken a terrible toll. In this land of plenty, too many Americans are suffering from over-nutrition that leads to poor nutrition.

Nurses, together with dietitians, physicians, exercise physiologists, and other health professionals can be effective educators and counselors for people who must lose weight and for those who want to lose weight. There is no such thing as a time-limited diet. To be effective, a sound dietary and exercise program must be a lifetime project. Unfortunately, many people believe that there is an easy and rapid way to lose weight.

Losing weight is hard work, but the greater challenge is lifetime weight control. Following a healthful and nutritious eating and exercise program is one of the most positive things a person can do. It leads to greater vitality and a longer life, certainly goals worth working for.

EXAM QUESTIONS

Chapter 11

Questions 93-100

93. Which of the following have been shown to increase chances of maintaining weight loss?

    a. "booster" sessions with the therapist 1 to 3 months apart
    b. review of weight loss strategies
    c. participation in bi-weekly peer support groups
    d. reading diet-related books

94. What is the most important reason to involve the patient's spouse and family in his or her diet program?

    a. they may be overweight as well and may need to use the same diet
    b. a diet can be easily sabotaged if the spouse or family doesn't understand its importance
    c. Yyou can learn more about the patient's diet habits from spouse and family
    d. the patient may be more open to diet suggestions

95. Some strategies to help prevent relapse include all of the following except:

    a. imagining a likely high-risk situation
    b. going out to a restaurant with a peer support group
    c. preplanning a binge
    d. allowing one uncontrolled binge weekly

96. How many individuals maintain weight loss over the long-term?

    a. very few
    b. about one-third
    c. about half
    d. about three-fourths

97. Which of the following best describes effective obesity treatment?

    a. obesity is a disease that can only be cured with caloric restriction and exercise
    b. obesity is a chronic disease that requires long-term treatment
    c. obesity results from faulty food behaviors which must be addressed during treatment
    d. the primary treatment for obesity is increased physical activity

98. All of the following are elements of a successful weight maintenance program except:

    a. setting realistic weight loss goals
    b. not expecting perfect adherence to diet
    c. exercising regularly
    d. adhering to a rigid diet

99. With therapist contact during the weight maintenance phase, which of the following topics is least important to focus on?

    a. learning food exchanges
    b. anticipating high-risk situations
    c. solving weight-related problems
    d. developing coping skills

100. Which is the best predictor of successful weight maintenance?

    a. successful experience with previous weight loss attempts
    b. being internally versus externally controlled
    c. having knowledge of calorie content of foods
    d. exercising regularly

APPENDIX A

RESOURCES

Organizations Offering Weight-related Materials

American Anorexia/Bulimia Association, Inc.
418 East 76th Street
New York, New York 10021
(212) 734-1114

American College of Sports Medicine
P.O. 1440
Indianapolis, Indiana 46206
(317) 637-9200

American Diabetes Association
Diabetes Information Service Center
1660 Duke Street
Alexandria, Virginia 22314
(1-800) 232-3472

American Dietetic Association
216 West Jackson Boulevard, Suite 800
Chicago, Illinois 60606-6995
(312) 899-0040

Bloomington Heart and Health Program
1900 West Old Shakopee Road
Bloomington, Minnesota 55431
(612) 887-9603

Bulimia Anorexia Self-Help
6125 Clayton Avenue, Suite 215
St. Louis, MO 63139
(1-800) 227-4785

Obesity Education Initiative
National Heart, Lung, and Blood Institute Programs
Information Center
P.O. Box 30105
Bethesda, Maryland 20824-0105
(301) 951-3260

Society for Nutrition Education
2001 Killebrew Drive
Suite 340
Minneapolis, Minnesota 55425-1882
(1-800) 235-6690

Other Specific Materials

Lifesteps (15-week weight loss program)
National Dairy Council
O'Hare International Center
10255 West Higgins Road
Rosemont, Illinois 60018-5616
(708) 803-2000

Obesity Update Newsletter
6900 Grove Road
Thorofare, New Jersey 08086-9864
(1-800) 257-8290

Learn Education Center
1555 West Mockingbird Lane
Suite 203
Dallas, Texas
(1-800) 736-7323:

> *The Learn Program for Weight Control* by Kelley
> D. Brownell
> American Health Publishing Co., 1991.

Living With Exercise by Steven N. Blair
American Health Publishing Co., 1991.

Weight Control Digest (bi-monthly newsletter)
Publication of Learn Education Center, Dallas,
Texas.

The Weight Maintenance Survival Guide by Kelly
D. Brownell and Judith Rodin
Brownell and Hager Publishing Co. 1990.

Shapedown (weight control program for children
and adolescents)
Balboa Publishing
11 Library Place
San Anselmo, California 94960
(415) 453-8886

APPENDIX B

Calorie and Fat Content of Some Fast Foods[*]

Arby's	Calories	Fat (grams)
chicken breast fillet	445	22.5
grilled chicken barbecue	386	13.1
fish fillet	526	27.0
ham n' cheese	355	14.2
roast beef sub	623	32.0
turkey sub	486	19.0
french fries	246	13.2
broccoli n' cheddar baked potato	417	17.9
garden salad, no dressing	117	5.2
chef salad, no dressing	205	9.5
light roast beef	294	10.0
light roast turkey deluxe	260	6.0
light roast chicken deluxe	276	7.0
old fashioned chicken noodle soup	99	1.8

Burger King		
whopper sandwich	570	31
cheeseburger	300	14
hamburger	260	10
BK broiler chicken sandwich	280	10
ocean catch fish fillet sandwich	450	28
chef salad, no dressing	178	9
side salad, no dressing	25	0
medium french fries	372	20

*   Based on nutritional information supplied by each food chain, Spring, 1993.

To determine the percentage of calories supplied by fat, multiply grams of fat by 9, divide by total calories in the food, and multiply by 100.

For example, if a food has 663 calories and 37 grams of fat:

1. $37 \times 9 = 333$ calories from fat
2.   (333 fat calories/663 total calories) $\times 100 = 50$ percent of calories from fat

Kentucky Fried Chicken

original recipe, center breast	260	14
original recipe, drumstick	152	9
extra crispy recipe, center breast	344	21
extra crispy recipe, drumstick	205	14
buttermilk biscuit	235	12
mashed potatoes and gravy	71	2
french fries	244	12
corn on the cob	90	2
coleslaw	114	6

McDonald's

hamburger	255	9
cheeseburger	305	13
quarter pounder	410	20
big mac	500	26
filet-o-fish	370	18
McChicken	415	20
chicken fajitas	185	8
small french fries	220	12
chicken McNuggets	270	15
chef salad, no dressing	170	9
side salad, no dressing	50	2

Rax

regular rax	262	10
deluxe roast beef	498	30
beef, bacon 'n cheddar	523	32
philly melt	396	16
grilled chicken breast sandwich	402	23
french fries	282	14
baked potato, plain	264	0

Taco Bell

taco	183	11
soft taco	225	12
tostada	243	11
taco supreme	230	15
bean burrito	387	14
beef burrito	431	21
combo burrito	407	16
nachos BellGrande	649	35
Mexican pizza	575	37
taco salad	905	61

<u>Wendy's</u>

plain single	340	15
Wendy's big classic	570	33
grilled chicken sandwich	340	13
fish fillet sandwich	460	25
small french fries	240	12
chili, regular, 9 ounce	220	7
baked potato, plain	270	0
baked potato, bacon and cheese	520	18

GLOSSARY

Adipose tissue connective tissue in which fat is stored and which has the cells distended by droplets of fat.

Aerobic exercise regular, rhythmic exercise that conditions the heart and lungs by improving oxygen consumption.

Alcohol an ingredient in beer, wine, liqueurs, cordials, and other distilled grain liquors. Pure alcohol provides seven calories per gram.

Atherosclerosis build-up of cholesterol and other fatty materials in the inner lining of the blood vessels, narrowing the vessels and making them less flexible.

Basal metabolic rate the energy necessary to support body functions at rest.

Behavior modification a method of restructuring behavior and environment to achieve a desired behavioral change.

Body mass index (BMI) weight in kilograms divided by height in meters squared.

Calorie a unit of measure that expresses the fuel or energy value of food.

Carbohydrate one of the three major macronutrients that provide calories. Carbohydrates provide four calories per gram.

> **complex carbohydrate** starch and dietary fiber
> **simple carbohydrate** naturally occurring and refined sugars

Cholesterol a fatlike substance in blood and other body compounds found only in animal foods. The body also manufactures cholesterol.

Exchange lists groups of foods categorized by their nutrient content. Foods in each exchange group have approximately the same nutrient content per portion and can be exchanged one for another.

Fat one of the three major macronutrients that provide calories. Fat is the most concentrated source of energy, providing nine calories per gram.

> **monounsaturated fat** fats with one double bond between carbon atoms. Monounsaturated fats tend to lower blood cholesterol levels.
> **omega-3 fat** a unique type of fat found in abundance in fish oil that may help protect against heart disease.
> **polyunsaturated fat** fats with two or more double bonds. Polyunsaturated fats also tend to lower blood cholesterol levels.
> **saturated fat** fats with no double bonds. Saturated fats raise blood cholesterol levels.

Fiber the undigestible portion of plant foods. Only plant foods provide fiber; animal foods provide no fiber.

> **insoluble fiber** fiber that does not dissolve in water. Insoluble fiber is found in wheat bran and most other cereal fibers. It gives bulk to the stool and helps prevent constipation.
> **soluble fiber** fiber that dissolves in water. Soluble fiber is found in dried beans and peas, oat products, and some fruits and vegetables. Soluble fiber helps lower blood cholesterol levels and stabilizes blood sugar levels.

Gastroplasty surgically stapling the stomach to restrict stomach size and capacity.

Hyperlipidemia a term for high blood cholesterol levels. Blood cholesterol levels under 200mg/dl are desirable. Levels between 220 and 239mg/dl are considered borderline high. Levels above 240mg/dl are considered high.

Hypertension high blood pressure, usually defined as a systolic blood pressure of 140mmHg or greater and/or diastolic blood pressure of 90mmHg or more.

Low-calorie diet (LCD) a diet providing about 1,000 to 1,500 calories daily to enable weight loss.

Minerals nutrients that are essential to the body in small amounts. Minerals are used to build and repair body tissue and control functions of the body.

Obesity a term used to describe excess body fat, usually defined as a weight greater than 20 percent over desirable body weight according to weight for height tables.

> **mild obesity** 20 to 40 percent over desirable weight
> **moderate obesity** 41 to 100 percent over desirable weight
> **morbid obesity** greater than 100 percent over desirable weight

Overweight a term used to describe individuals who weigh more than desirable according to weight for height tables but who may not necessarily be overfat. Overweight describes individuals who weigh up to 19 percent over desirable weight.

Protein one of the three major macronutrients that provide calories. Protein provides four calories per gram. Animal foods such as milk, meat, poultry, and fish provide high-quality complete protein; plant foods provide smaller amounts of protein, which must be combined to yield complete protein.

Recommended dietary allowances (RDA) standards of daily nutrient intake that are judged to meet the needs of most healthy persons. The Food and Nutrition Board of the National Academy of Sciences set these standards and revises them periodically.

Relapse loss of control over eating after weight loss, which could lead to weight regain.

Relative weight a patient's current weight in pounds as a percentage of desirable body weight listed in weight for height tables.

Thermic effect of food the energy necessary to digest food and drink.

Very low-calorie diet (VLCD) a severely restricted diet providing 600 to 800 calories daily, primarily of high-quality protein, supplemented with vitamins and minerals.

Vitamins nutrients essential to the body to assist in body processes and functions.

Weight cycling repeated cycles of weight loss followed by weight gain.

BIBLIOGRAPHY

Abraham, S., Collins, G., and Nordsieck, L. (1971). Relationship of childhood weight status to morbidity in adults. *HSMHA Health Reports*, 86, 273384.

American College of Sports Medicine. (1991). *Guidelines for exercise testing and prescription* (4th ed.). Philadelphia: Lea and Febiger.

American Diabetes Association. (1992). Nutrition recommendations and principles for individuals with diabetes mellitus. *Diabetes Care* 15, 21–28.

The American Diabetes and Dietetic Associations. (1988). *Eating Healthy Foods*. Alexandria, VA: The American Diabetes Association, Chicago, IL: The American Dietetic Association.

The American Diabetes and Dietetic Associations. (1989). *Exchange Lists for Weight Management*. Alexandria, VA: The American Diabetes Association, Chicago, IL: The American Dietetic Association.

American Dietetic Association. (1989). Position of the American Dietetic Association: Optimal weight as a health promotion strategy. *Journal of the American Dietetic Association* 89, 1814–17.

American Heart Association. (1987). *1987 heart facts*. Dallas, TX: American Heart Association.

American Heart Association (1987). *Designing a More Prudent Diet*.

Anderson, J.W. & Gustafson, N.J. (1987). Dietary fiber in disease prevention and treatment. *Comprehensive Therapy* 13, 43–53.

Anderson, J.W. & Gustafson, N.J. (1988). Hypocholesterolemic effects of oat and bean products. *American Journal of Clinical Nutrition* 48 (suppl), 749S–753S.

Andres, R. D., Elahi, J., Tobin, D., et al. (1985). Impact of age on weight goals. *Annals of Internal Medicine*, 103, 1030–1033.

Angel, A. (1978). Pathophysiologic changes in obesity. *Canadian Medical Association Journal*, 119(12), 1401–1406.

Aronow, W. S. (1980). Effect of non-nicotine cigarettes on carbon monoxide on angina. *Circulation*, 61, 262–265.

Ashley, F. & Kannel, W. (1974). Relation of weight change to changes in atherogenic traits: The Framingham Study. *Journal of Chronic Diseases* 27, 103–114.

Atkinson, R.L. (1989). Low and very low calorie diets. *Medical Clinics of North America* 73, 203–215.

Ballor, D.L., McCarthy, J.P., & Wilterdink, E.J. (1990). Exercise intensity does not affect composition of diet- and exercise-induced body mass loss. *American Journal of Clinical Nutrition* 51, 142–46.

Bierman, E. & Brunzell, J.D. (1992). Obesity and atherosclerosis. In P. Bjorntorp & B.N. Brodoff (Eds.), *Obesity* (pp.512–516). Philadelphia: J.B. Lippincott Co.

Bjorntorp, P. (1991). Metabolic implications of body fat distribution. *Diabetes Care* 14, 1132–43.

Bjorvell, H. & Rossner, S. (1992). A ten year follow-up of weight change in severely obese subjects treated in a behavioral modification program. *International Journal of Obesity* 16, 623–625.

Blackburn, G.L. & Kanders, B.S. (1987). Medical evaluation and treatment of the obese patient with cardiovascular disease. *American Journal of Cardiology* 60, 55G–58G.

Blundell, J.E. (1990). Appetite disturbance and the problems of overweight. *Drugs* 39(Suppl 3), 1–19.

Bonadonna, R.C. & DeFronzo, R.A. (1992). Glucose metabolism in obesity and type II diabetes. In P. Bjorntorp & B.N. Brodoff, (Eds.), *Obesity* (pp. 474–501). Philadelphia: J.B. Lippincott Co.

Bowen, D.J., Tomoyasu, N. & Cauce, A.M. (1991). The triple threat: a discussion of gender, class, and race difference in weight. *Women's Health* 17, 123–43.

Bray, G. A. (1976). *The obese patient: Major problems in internal medicine.* Philadelphia: W. B. Saunders Company.

Bray, G. A. (1979). Obesity in America: An overview of the Second Fogarty International Center Conference on Obesity. *International Journal of Obesity*, 3, 363–375.

Bray, G.A. (1985a). Complications of obesity. *Annals of Internal Medicine* 103, 1052–62.

Bray, G. A. (1985b). Obesity: Definition, diagnosis, and disadvantages. *Austrian Journal of Medicine*, 142 (Suppl. 7), S2–S8.

Bray, G.A. (1990). Exercise and obesity. In C. Bouchard, R.J. Shepard, T. Stephans, et. al. (Eds.), *Exercise, fitness, and health*, (pp.497–510). Chapaign, IL: Human Kinetics.

Bray, G. (1992a). Pathophysiology of obesity. *American Journal of Clinical Nutrition* 55 (suppl), 488S–494S.

Bray, G. (1992b). Obesity: Historical development of scientific and cultural ideals. In P. Bjorntorp & B.N. Brodoff, (Eds.). *Obesity*, (pp. 281–293). Philadelphia: J.B. Lippincott Co.

Brown, P. J., Konner, M. (1987). An anthropological perspective on obesity. *Annals of the New York Academy of Science*, 499, 29–46.

Brownell, K.D. (1983). The contribution of psychological and behavioral factors to a classification scheme for obesity. In J. Hirsch & T.B. Van Itallie, (Eds.), *Recent advances in obesity research, proceedings of the 4th international congress on obesity*, (pp. 150–154). London, England: John Libbey.

Brownell, K.D. (1992). Relapses and the treatment of obesity. In T.A. Wadden & Van Itallie, T.B. (Eds.), *Treatment of the Seriously Obese Patient.*, (pp.437–55). New York: The Guildford Press.

Brownell, K.D. & Stunkard, A.J. (1980). Physical activity in the development and control of obesity. In. A.L. Stunkard (Ed.), *Obesity*, (pp.300–324). Philadelphia: Saunders.

Bruch, H. (1978). *The golden cage: The enigma of anorexia nervosa.* New York: Random House.

Bruch, H. (1979). *Eating disorders: Obesity, anorexia nervosa, and the person within.* New York: Basic Books.

Build and Blood Pressure Study. (1959). Chicago: *Society of Actuaries*.

Butrum, R.R., Clifford, C.K. & Lanza E. (1988). NCI dietary guidelines: Rationale. *American Journal of Clinical Nutrition* 48, 888–891.

Callaway, C.W. & Pemberton, C. (1985). Relationship of basal metabolic rates to meal-eating patterns. In: J. Hirsch & T.B. Van Itallie, (Eds.), *Recent advances in obesity research.* *Proceedings of the 4th International Congress on Obesity,* (pp. 50A). London: Libbey.

Case, R.B., Heller, S.S., Case, N.B., et. al. (1985). Multicenter Post-Infraction Research Group: Type A behavior and survival after acute myocardial infarction. *New England Journal of Medicine* 312, 737–741.

Centers for Disease Control. (1991). Leads from the "Morbidity and Mortality Weekly Report." *Journal of the American Medical Association* 266, 2811–12.

Christakis, G. (1979). How to make a nutritional diagnosis without really trying. A. Adult nutritional diagnosis. *Journal of the Florida Medical Association,* 66, 349–356.

Connor, S. L., & Connor, W. E. (1986). *The New American Diet.* New York: Simon and Schuster.

Danish, S. J., Lang, D., Smiciklas-Wright, H., et al. (1968). Nutrition counseling skills. Continuing education for the dietitian. *Topics in Clinical Nutrition,* 1, 25–32.

DeFronzo, R.A. & Ferrannini, E. (1991). Insulin resistance: A multifaceted syndrome responsible for NIDDM, obesity, hypertension, dyslipidemia, and atherosclerotic cardiovascular disease. *Diabetes Care* 14, 173–94.

Despres, J.P., Moorjani, S., Lupien, P.J. et al. (1990). Regional distribution of body fat, plasma, lipoproteins, and cardiovascular disease. *Arteriosclerosis* 10, 497–511.

de Zwaan, M., Nutzinger, D.O. & Schoenbeck, G. (1992). Binge eating in overweight women. *Comprehensive Psychiatry* 33, 256–61.

Dietz, W. (1992). Childhood obesity. In P. Bjorntorp & B.N. Brodoff (Eds.). *Obesity,* (pp.606–609). Philadelphia: J.B. Lippincott Co.

Drenick, E. J., Bale, F. S., Seltzer, A., et al. (1980). Excess mortality and causes of death in morbidly obese men. *Journal of the American Medical Association,* 243, 445.

Duncan, J.J., Gordon, N.F. & Scott, C.B. (1991). Women walking for health and fitness: How much is enough? *Journal of the American Medical Association* 266, 3295–3299.

Dwyer, J.T. (1992). Treatment of obesity: Conventional programs and fad diets. In P. Bjorntorp & B.N. Brodoff, (Eds.). *Obesity,* (pp. 662–667). Philadelphia: J.B. Lippincott Co.

Eckel, R.H. (1992). Insulin resistance: and adaptation for weight maintenance. *Lancet.* 340, 1452–1453.

Eliahou, H.E., Shechter, P. & Blare, A. Hypertension in obesity. In P. Bjorntorp & B.N. Brodoff, (Eds). *Obesity* (pp. 532–39). Philadelphia: J.B. Lippincott Co.

Enos, W. F., Holmes, R. H., & Beyer, J. (1953). Coronary disease among United States soldiers killed in Korea. *Journal of the American Medical Association,* 152, 1090–1093.

Everhart, J.E., Pettitt, D.J. & Bennett, P.H. (1992). Duration of obesity increases the incidence of NIDDM. *Diabetes* 41, 235–240.

Farley, D. (1992). Eating disorders require medical attention. *FDA Consumer* March, 27–29.

Ferguson, S. (1983). The diet center program: Lose weight fast and keep it off forever. Boston, Toronto: Little, Brown, and Co.

Food and Nutrition Board of the National Academy of Sciences, National Research Council. (1989). *Recommended Dietary Allowances,* (10th ed.). Washington, D.C.: National Academy Press.

Foss, M. L. (1984). Exercise concerns and precautions for the obese. In J. Storlie & H.A. Jordan, (Eds.), *Nutrition and exercise in obesity management* (pp. 123–148). New York: Spectrum Books.

Fox, K.P. (1992). A clinical approach to exercise in the markedly obese. In T.A. Wadden T.B. Van Itallie, (Eds.). *Treatment of the Seriously Obese Patient,* (pp. 354–82). New York: The Guildford Press.

Frankle, R.T. (1987). "Weight Control for the Adult and Elderly" In R.T. Frankel & M.U. Yang (Eds.). *Obesity and Weight Control,* (pp. 361–89). Rockville, MD: Aspen Publishers Inc.

Friedman, G. D., Kannel, W. B., and Dawber, R. R. (1966). The epidemiology of gallbladder disease: Observations in the Framingham study. *Journal of Chronic Disease,* 19, 273–292.

Frohlich, E. D. (1983). Hypertension and hypertensive heart disease. In E. K. Chung (Ed.), *Quick reference to cardiovascular diseases (2nd ed),* (pp. 175–187). Philadelphia: J. P. Lippincott.

Garfinkel, L. (1985). Overweight and cancer. *Annals of Internal Medicine* 103, 1034.

Gilbert, S. (1975). *Fat free common sense for young weight worriers.* New York: Macmillan.

Goldstein, D.J. (1992). Beneficial health effects of modest weight loss. *International Journal of Obesity* 16, 397–415.

Goodhart, R. S., & Shils, M. E. (Eds). (1980). *Modern nutrition in health and disease.* Philadelphia: Lea & Febiger.

Gortmaker, S.L., Dietz, W.H., Sobol, A.M., et. al. (1987). Increasing pediatric obesity in the United States. *American Journal of Diseases of Children* 141, 535.

Graber, A., Christman, B., Alonga, M., et al. (1977). Evaluation of the diabetic patient education programs. *Diabetes* 26, 1: 61–64.

Grilo, C.M., & Brownell, K.D. (1993) "Relapse: Why,How, and What to Do About It." *Weight Control Digest* vol 1. No. 3; 217–232.

Grommet, J.K. (1988). "Assessment of the Obese Person." In R.T. Frankle and M.U. Yang, (Eds.), *Obesity and Weight Control: The Health Professional's Guide to Understanding and Treatment* , (pp.111–132). Rockville, MD.: Aspen Publishers, Inc.

Grundy, S. M. (1983). Atherosclerosis: Pathology, pathogenesis, and role of risk factors. *Disease-a-Month,* June, 3–58.

Grundy, S. M., Greenland, P., Herd, A., et al. (1987). Cardiovascular and risk factor evaluation of healthy American adults: A statement for physicians by an ad hoc committee appointed by the steering committee. *Circulation,* 75, 1339A-1362A.

Grundy, S.M. & Barneltt, J.P. (1990). Metabolic and health complications of obesity. In. R.C. Bone, (Ed.). *Disease-a-month,* (vol. 36 pg.643–731) St. Louis: C.V. Mosby Year Book.

Gustafson-Larson, A.M. & Terry, R.D. (1992). Weight-related behaviors and concerns of fourth-grade children. *Journal of the American Dietetic Association* 92, 818–822.

Guthrie, H. (1988). Nutrition for the elderly. In B. Lipsitz (Ed.), *Nutrition for the elderly, symposium II.* New York: Raven Press.

Guy-Grand, B. (1992). Long-term pharmacological treatment of obesity. In T.A. Wadden & T.B. Van Itallie, T B. (Eds.). *Treatment of the Seriously Obese Patient*, (pp. 478–95). New York: The Guildford Press.

Gwinup, G. (1970). *Energetics: Your key to weight control.* Los Angeles: Sherbourne Press.

House of Representatives (1990). *Deception and Fraud in the Diet Industry Part II.* Hearing before the Subcommittee on Regulation, Business Opportunities, and Energy of the Committee on Small Business. Serial No. 101–57.

Hubert, H. B., Feinlieb, M., McNamara, I. I., et al. (1983). Obesity as an independent risk factor for heart disease: A 26-year follow-up of participants in the Framingham heart study. *Circulation*, 67, 968–977.

Hypertension Detection and Follow-up Program Cooperative Group. (1979). Five-year follow-up findings of the hypertension detection and follow-up program. *Journal of the American Medical Association*, 242, 2562.

Jeffrey, R., Wing, R., & French, S. (1992). Weight cycling and cardiovascular disease risk factors in obese men and women. *American Journal of Clinical Nutrition* 55, 641–644.

Jequier, E., Felber, J. P. (1987). Indirect calorimetry. *Baillieres Cliniques Endocrinologie et Metabolism*, 1(4), 911–935.

Jequier, E. (1990). Energy metabolism in obese patients before and after weight loss, and in patients who have relapsed. *International Journal of Obesity* 14(suppl 1), 59–67.

Johnston, F.E. (1985). Health implications of childhood obesity. *Annals of Internal Medicine* 103, 1068.

Kahn, H.S., Williamson, D.F. & Stevens, J.A. (1991). Race and weight change in US women: The roles of socioeconomic marital status. *American Journal of Public Health* 81, 319–323.

Kannel, W. B. (1986). Epidemiologic insights into atherosclerotic cardiovascular disease from the Framingham study. In M.L. Pollock & D. H. Schmidt (Eds.), *Heart disease and rehabilitation (2nd ed.)*, (pp. 3–28). New York: John Wiley & Sons.

Kato, I., Nomura, A., Stemmetmann, G.N., et. al. (1992). Prospective study of clinical gallbladder disease and its association with obesity, physical activity, and other factors. *Digestive Diseases and Sciences* 37, 784–90.

Kayman, S., Bruvold, W. & Stern, J.S. (1990). Maintenance and relapse after weight loss in women: behavioral aspects. *American Journal of Clinical Nutrition* 52, 800–807.

Keesey, R. E. (1988). The body-weight set point. What can you tell your patients? *Postgraduate Medicine*, 83, 114–127.

Kral, J.G. (1992). Surgical treatment of obesity. In T.A. Wadden & T.B. Van Itallie, (Eds.). *Treatment of the Seriously Obese Patient*, (pp. 496–506). New York: The Guildford Press.

Kumanyika, S. (1987). Obesity in black women. *Epidemiology Review* 31–50.

Lantingua, R.A., Amatruda, J.A., Biddle, T.L., et. al. (1980). Cardiac arrhythmias associated with a liquid protein diet for the treatment of obesity. *New England Journal of Medicine* 303, 735–38.

Lanzola, A., Tagliabue, G., Bozzi, G., et. al. (1991). Obesity, diet, and body temperature. *Annals of Nutrition and Metabolism* 35, 274–283.

Lapidus, L., Bentgsson, C., Larsson, B., et al. (1984). Distribution of adipose tissue and risk of cardiovascular disease and death: 12-year follow-up of participants in the population study of Gothenborg, Sweden. *British Medical Journal*, 289, 1257–1261.

Lee, I.M. & Paffenbarger, R.S. Jr. (1992). Quetelet's index and risk of colon cancer in college alumni. *Journal of the National Cancer Institute* 84, 1326–31.

Lew, E. A., and Garfinkle, L. (1979). Variations in mortality by weight among 750,000 men and women. Journal of Chronic Diseases 32, 563-576.

Lichtman, S.W., Pisarska, K., Berman, E.R., et. al. (1992). Discrepancy between self-reported and actual calorie intake and exercise in obese subjects. *New England Journal of Medicine* 327, 1893–98.

Lissner, L., Odell, P. & D'Agostino, R. (1991). Variability of body weight and health outcomes in the Framingham population. *New England Journal of Medicine* 324, 1839–1844.

Logue, A. W., Pena-Correal, T. E., Rodriquex, M. L., et al. (1986). Self-control in adult humans: Variations in positive reinforcer amount and delay. *Journal of the Experimental Analysis of Behavior*, 46, 159–173.

Mattila, K., Haavisto, M. & Rajala, R. (1986). Body mass index and mortality in the elderly. *British Medical Journal* 292, 867–868

McGinnis, J.M. & Ballard–Barbash, R.M. (1991). Obesity in minority populations: Policy implications of research. *American Journal of Clinical Nutrition* 91, 1512S–1514S.

Manson, J.E., Colditz, G.A., Stampfer, M.J., et. al. (1990). A prospective study of obesity and risk of coronary heart disease in women. *New England Journal of Medicine* 322,882–889.

Mayer, J., Marshall, N. B., Vitale, J. J., et al. (1954). Exercise, food intake, and body weight in normal rats and genetically obese adult mice. *American Journal of Physiology*, 177, 544–548.

Mendelson, B. K., White, D. R. (1982). Relation between body-esteem and self-esteem of obese and normal children. *Perceptual and Motor Skills*, 54(3), 899–905.

Metropolitan Life Insurance Company (1982). Metropolitan height and weight tables. *Metropolitan Life Insurance Company Statistical Bulletin*, 64, 1–9.

Must, A., Jacques, P.F., Dallal, G.E., et. al. (1989). Long-term morbidity and mortality of overweight adolescents: A follow-up of the Harvard Growth Study of 1922 to 1935. *New England Journal of Medicine* 327, 1350–1355.

National Center for Health Statistics. (1986). Prevalence, impact, and impact of known diabetes in the United States. In Advance data from vital health statistics, *U.S. Department of Health and Human Services* publication no. 86-1250. Hyattsville, MD: U.S. Public Health Service.

National Center for Health Statistics. (1987). Najjar, M.F. & Rowland, M. Anthropometric reference data and prevalence of overweight, United States, 1976–80. *Vital Health Statistics* 238 (11), 1–73.

National Center for Health Statistics. (1989). Najjar, M.F. & Kuczmarski, R.J. Anthropometric data and prevalence of overweight for Hispanics: 1882–84. *Vital Health Statistics* 239 (11), 1–106.

National Cholesterol Education Program, National Institutes of Health. (1989). *Report of the Expert Panel on Detection, Evaluation, and Treatment of High Blood Cholesterol in Adults.* Washington, D.C.: U.S. Government Printing Office. NIH Publication No. 89–2925.

National Heart, Lung, and Blood Institute, National Institutes of Health. (1993). *Data Fact Sheet: Obesity and Cardiovascular Disease.* Washington, D.C.: U.S. Government Printing Office.

National Heart, Lung, and Blood Institute, National Institutes of Health. (1990). *Infomemo* Spring.

National Institutes of Health. (1985). "National Institutes of Health Consensus Development Panel on the Health Implications of Obesity: National Institutes of Health Consensus Development Conference Statement" *Annals of Internal Medicine* 103, 1073–77.

National Institutes of Health (1987). *Gallbladder Disease.* Bethesda., MD.

National Institutes of Health. (1993). *The fifth report of the Joint National Committee on Detection, Evaluation, and Treatment of High Blood Pressure.* Washington, D.C.: U.S. Government Printing Office. NIH Publication No. 93–1088.

National Institutes of Health Technology Assessment Conference. (1992). Methods for voluntary weight loss and control. *Annals of Internal Medicine* 116, 942–949.

National Research Council. (1989). *Diet and health: Implications for reducing chronic disease risk.* Washington, D.C.: National Academy Press.

Obesity Update Newsletter (1993). Winter. Thorofare, New Jersey.

Paffenbarger, R.S., Hyde, R.T., Wing, A.L., et. al. (1993). The association of changes in physical-activity level and other lifestyle characteristics with mortality among men. *New England Journal of Medicine* 328, 358–45.

Pemberton, C. (1984). "Clinical Assessment of the Obese Individual." In J. Storlie & H.A. Jordan, (Eds.). *Evaluation and Treatment of Obesity,* (pp.71–92). Champaign, IL.: Life Enhancement Publications.

Perkins, K.A., Epstein, L.H., Stiller, R.L., et. al. (1989). Acute effects of nicotine on resting metabolic rate in cigarette smokers. *American Journal of Clinical Nutrition* 50, 545–550.

Perri, M.G. (1992). Improving maintenance of weight loss following treatment by diet and lifestyle modification. In Wadden, T.A. and Van Itallie, T.B. (Eds.). *Treatment of the seriously obese patient.* (pp. 456–77). New York: The Guildford Press.

Perri, M.G., Nezv, A.M. & Viegener, B.J. (1992). *Improving the long-term management of obesity.* New York: John Wiley and Sons.

Perri, M.G., Sears, S.F. Jr & Clark, J.E. (1993). Strategies for improving maintenance of weight loss: Toward a continuing care model of obesity management. *Diabetes Care* 16, 200–09.

Peternelj-Taylor, C.A. (1989). The effects of patient weight and sex on nurses' perceptions: a proposed model of nurse withdrawal. *Journal of Advances in Nursing* 14, 744–54.

Podell, R. N., & Stewart, M. M. (Eds.). (1983). *Primary prevention of coronary heart disease.* Menlo Park, CA: Addison-Wesley Publishing Company.

Poehlman, E.T. (1986). Genotype-controlled changes in body composition and fat morphology following overfeeding in twins. *American Journal of Clinical Nutrition* 43, 723–731.

Posner, Barbara M. (1979). *Nutrition and the Elderly.* Toronto: D. C. Heath and Company.

Price, R.A., Stunkard, A.J. (1989). Commingling analysis of obesity in twins. *Human Heredity* 39, 121–35.

Ravussin, E. (1993). Energy metabolism in obesity: Studies in the Pima Indians. *Diabetes Care* 16, 232–238.

Ravussin, E. & Bogardus, C. (1992). A brief overview of human energy metabolism and its relationship to essential obesity. *American Journal of Clinical Nutrition* 55, 242S–245S.

Ravussin, E., Lillioja, S., Knowler, W.C., et. al. (1988). Reduced rate of energy expenditure as a risk factor for body-weight gain. *New England Journal of Medicine* 318, 467–72.

Roberts, S.B., Savage, J., Coward, W.A., et. al. (1988). Energy expenditure and intake in infants born to lean and overweight mothers. *New England Journal of Medicine* 318, 461–466.

Robison, J., Hoerr, S.L., Strandmark, J., et. al. (1993). Obesity, weight loss, and health. *Journal of the American Dietetic Association* 93, 445–449.

Rossouw, J.E., Lewis, B. & Rifkind, B.M. (1990). The value of lowering cholesterol after myocardial infarction. *New England Journal of Medicine* Oct 18, 1112–13.

Roubenoff, R., Klag, M.J. & Mead, L.A., et. al. Incidence and risk factors for gout in white men. *Journal of the American Medical Association* 266, 3004–7.

Sandvik, L., Erikssen, J., Thaulow, E., et. al. (1993). Physical Fitness as a Predictor of Mortality Among Healthy, Middle-Aged Norwegian Men. *New England Journal of Medicine* 328, 533–37.

Savage, P.J. & Harlan, W.R. (1991). Racial and ethnic diversity in obesity and other risk factors cardiovascular disease: Implications for studies and treatment. *Ethnic Diseases* 1, 200–211.

Schachter, S. (1971). Some extraordinary facts about obese humans and rats. *American Journal of Psychology*, 26, 129–144.

Schapiru, D.V., Kimar, N.B. & Lyman, G.H., et. al. (1990). Abdominal obesity and breast cancer risks. *Annals of Internal Medicine* 112, 182–186.

Schauer, P.R., Ramos, R. & Ghiatas, A.A., et. al. (1992). Virulent diverticular disease in young obese men. *American Journal of Surgery* 164, 443–46.

Sclafani, A., Springer, D (1985). Dietary obesity in adult rats: similarities to hypothalamic and human obesity syndrome. *Physiology & Behavior* 17, 461–471.

Sharp, J. T., Barrocas, M., & Chokroverty, S. (1983). The cardiorespiratory effects of obesity on respiratory function. *American Review of Respiratory Disease*, 128, 501–506.

Sherry, B., Springer, D.A. & Connell, F.A., et. al. (1992). Short, thin, or obese?: Comparing growth indexes of children from high- and low-poverty areas. *Journal of the American Dietetic Association* 92, 1092–95.

Simonson, M., & Heilman, J. R. (1983). *The Complete University Medical Diet.* New York: Rawson Associates.

Sjostrom, L. (1992). Mortality of severely obese subjects. *American Journal of Clinical Nutrition* 55(suppl), 516S–523S.

Skelton, N.K. & Skelton, W.P. (1992). Medical implications of obesity: Losing pounds, gaining years. *Postgraduate Medicine* 151–156, 159–162.

Smoller, J.W., Wadden, T.A. & Brownell, K.D. (1988). "Popular and very low-calorie diets in the treatment of obesity." In R.T. Frankle & M.V. Yang, (Eds.). *Obesity and Weight Control: The Health Professional's Guide to Understanding and Treatment,* (pp.133–164). Rockville, MD: Aspen Publishers, Inc.

Society of Actuaries and Association of Life Insurance Medical Directors of America. (1980). *Build Study of 1979.* Chicago, IL: Society of Actuaries.

Spitzer, R. L., Endicott, J., and Robbins, E. (1975). *Research Diagnostic Criteria (RDC) for a Selected Group of Functional Disorders.* 2nd ed. Biometrics Research, New York State Psychiatric Institute, New York.

Stein, R.F. (1987). Comparison of self-concept of non-obese and obese university junior female nursing students. *Adolescence* 22, 77–90.

Stein, J. S., & Lowney, T. (1986). Obesity: The role of physical activity. In K. D. Brownell & J. T. Foreyt (Eds.), *Handbook of early disorders* (pp. 145–158). New York: Basic Books.

Stuart, R. B., & Davis, B. (1972). *Slim chance in a fat world: Behavioral control of obesity.* Champaign, IL: Research Press.

Stunkard, A. J. (1980). *Obesity.* Philadelphia: W. B. Saunders Company.

Stunkard, A.J. (1986). A study of human obesity. *Journal of the American Medical Association* 256, 51–54.

Stunkard, A.J. (1992). An overview of current treatment for obesity. In T.A. Wadden & T.B. Van Itallie, (Eds.). *Treatment of the Seriously Obese Patient.* New York: The Guildford Press.

Stunkard, A. J. & Stellar, E. (Eds.). (1984). *Eating and its disorders.* New York: Raven Press.

Sturdevant, R. A., Pearce, L., Dayton, S. (1973). Increased prevalence of cholelithiasis in men ingesting a severe cholesterol-lowering diet. *New England Journal of Medicine* 288, 2427.

The Surgeon General's report on nutrition and health (1988). *U.S. Department of Health and Human Services.* DHHS (PHS) Publication No. 88–50210. Washington, D.C.: U.S. Government Printing Office.

Toeller, M., Gries, F. A., & Dannehl, K. (1982). Natural history of glucose intolerance in obesity: A 10-year observation. *International Journal of Obesity,* 6 (Suppl. 1), 145–149.

Tremblay, A., Despres, J.P., Maheux, J., et. al. (1991). *Medical Science Sports and Exercise* 23, 1326–1331.

Tuck, M. L., Sowers, L., Dornfield, G., et al. (1981). The effect of weight reduction on blood pressure, plasma renin activity, and plasma aldosterone levels in obese patients. *New England Journal of Medicine* 304, 933–945.

U.S. Department of Agriculture and Health and Human Services. (1990). *Nutrition and your health: Dietary guidelines for Americans,* (3rd ed.). Washington, D.C.: U.S. Government Printing Office.

U.S. Department of Agriculture, Human Nutrition Information Service. (1992). *Food guide pyramid: A guide to daily food choices*, Leaflet No. 572. Washington, D.C.: U.S. Government Printing Office.

Van Dale, D., Saris, W.H.M. & ten Hoor, F. (1990). Weight maintenance and resting metabolic rage 18–40 months after a diet/exercise treatment. *International Journal of Obesity* 14, 347–60.

Van Itallie, T.B. (1979). Obesity: adverse effects on health and longevity. *American Journal of Clinical Nutrition* 32, 2723–33.

Van Itallie, T.B. (1992). Body weight: Morbidity and longevity. In P. Bjorntorp & B.N. Brodoff, (Eds.). *Obesity,* (pp. 361–369). Philadelphia: J.B. Lippincott Co.

Waaler, H. T. (1983). Weight and mortality: The Norwegian experience. *Acta Medica Scandinavica* 649, 1–55.

Wadden, T.A., Sternberg, A.J., Letizia K.A., et. al. (1989). Treatment of obesity by very low calorie diet, behavior therapy, and their combination: A five–year perspective. *International Journal of Obesity* 13, 39–46.

Wadden, T. A., and Stunkard, A. J. (1986). A controlled trial of very-low calorie diet, behavior therapy, and their combination in the treatment of obesity. *Journal of Consultations in Clinical Psychology* 54, 482–488.

Wadden, T.A., Stunkard, A.J. & Brownell, K.D. (1993): Very low calorie diets: Their efficiency, safety, and future. *Annals of Internal Medicine* 99, 675–84.

Walberg-Rankin, J. (1992). Utilizing exercise in the treatment of obesity. *Comprehensive Therapy* 18, 31–34.

Willard, M.D. (1991). Obesity: types and treatments. *American Family Physician* 43, 2099–108.

Williams, B. J., Martin, S., & Foreyt, J. P. (Eds). (1976). *Obesity: Behavioral approaches to dietary management.* New York: Brunner/Mazel.

Winick, M. (1985). *Your personalized health profile: Choosing the diet that's right for you.* New York: William Morrow and Company.

INDEX

LIFETIME WEIGHT CONTROL PRE-TEST ANSWER KEY

1.	a	Chapter 1
2.	b	Chapter 1
3.	c	Chapter 1
4.	c	Chapter 2
5.	d	Chapter 2
6.	b	Chapter 3
7.	d	Chapter 3
8.	a	Chapter 4
9.	d	Chapter4
10.	d	Chapter 5
11.	d	Chapter 5
12.	a	Chapter 5
13.	a	Chapter 6
14.	b	Chapter 6
15.	b	Chapter 7
16.	a	Chapter 7
17.	c	Chapter 8
18.	d	Chapter 8
19.	a	Chapter 8
20.	b	Chapter 9
21.	b	Chapter 9
22.	b	Chapter 10
23.	a	Chapter 10
24.	b	Chapter 11
25.	d	Chapter 11

NOTES

NOTES